Psychology Revivals

Psychology and Religion

Originally published in 1963, this book states that religion is a universal phenomenon and a dominant factor in human development. It must therefore be studied psychologically as a primordial aspect of human consciousness. This involves a balanced presentation of anthropology, comparative religion, evolution and the theories of those considered at the time the three greatest psychologists of the twentieth century, William James, Sigmund Freud and C. G. Jung.

This book is a highly readable study of the psychology of religion in the twentieth century. The first part is devoted to a clear exposition of modern theories of the time, particularly those of Freud and Jung, and the second part is a comprehensive study of the way in which such theories help to elucidate religious practices and the phenomena of religious experience and mysticism.

It assumes that Freudian theories are capable of a positive interpretation and that the Jungian theories of archetypes and symbolism furnish one of the most brilliant explanations of religious phenomena. The section which deals with myth and historical religion is a positive contribution to what was often regarded, theologically, as a contentious issue.

Psychology and Religion

An Introduction to Contemporary Views

G. Stephens Spinks

Routledge
Taylor & Francis Group

First published in 1963
by Methuen & Co. Ltd

This edition first published in 2026 by Routledge
4 Park Square, Milton Park, Abingdon, Oxon, OX14 4RN

and by Routledge
605 Third Avenue, New York, NY 10158

Routledge is an imprint of the Taylor & Francis Group, an informa business

Publisher's Note

The publisher has gone to great lengths to ensure the quality of this reprint but points out that some imperfections in the original copies may be apparent.

Disclaimer

The publisher has made every effort to trace copyright holders and welcomes correspondence from those they have been unable to contact.

For Product Safety Concerns and Information please contact our EU representative GPSR@taylorandfrancis.com. Taylor & Francis Verlag GmbH, Kaufingerstraße 24, 80331 München, Germany

A Library of Congress record exists under LCCN: 63025298

ISBN: 978-1-041-24251-2 (hbk)
ISBN: 978-1-003-74095-7 (ebk)
ISBN: 978-1-041-24259-8 (pbk)

Book DOI 10.4324/9781003740957

Psychology and Religion

AN INTRODUCTION TO CONTEMPORARY VIEWS

BY

G. STEPHENS SPINKS

M.A, Ph.D.

One-time Editor of the Hibbert Journal and Upton Lecturer in the Psychology of Religion, Oxford

METHUEN & CO LTD

36 Essex Street · London WC2

First published in 1963

Printed in Great Britain by
Butler & Tanner Ltd
Frome and London
Catalogue No. 2/2595/10

To

two medical friends

R. A. N. and M. K. S.

CONTENTS

Part II. Psychology and Religious Practices

ACKNOWLEDGEMENTS

My thanks are due to The Hogarth Press Limited for permission to quote from *The Future of an Illusion*, *The Ego and the Id*, *Moses and Monotheism*, and *Group Psychology and the Analysis of the Ego* by Freud; to Messrs Routledge and Kegan Paul Limited for permission to quote from *Totem and Taboo* by Freud; and to the Bollingen Foundation and Messrs Routledge and Kegan Paul Limited for permission to quote from *Modern Man in Search of a Soul*, *Collected Works*, volumes 7, 8 and 11, *Contributions to Analytical Psychology*, *Integration of the Personality*, *Freud and Psycho-Analysis*, and *Psychological Types* by Jung.

I am grateful to the Reverend Roger Thomas, M.A., Dr. Williams's Librarian, for the services of the Library and his assistance in checking details in the Bibliography; and to Miss M. Beadle, B.Sc., for reading the proofs.

I have endeavoured to acknowledge both in text and bibliography the numerous authors whose works I have consulted, and from whom I have made quotations and borrowed material. But there is always a possibility that some acknowledgement may not have been made. The mind is fed by many streams, the sources of which are not always remembered or even known but whose contributions are a matter for grateful appreciation by all who profit from them.

G. S. S.

PREFACE

When William James delivered his Gifford lectures on *The Varieties of Religious Experience* (1901–1902), he not only made the most outstanding of all single contributions to the psychology of religion, but also set the pattern for the majority of subsequent studies during the next half-century. The influence of the *Varieties* is such that even today few are able to write on this subject without making generous use both of the actual text and of James's ideas. Indeed, writers whose works have been most conspicuously appreciated in the English-speaking world – such as J. Bissett Pratt, R. H. Thouless and L. W. Grensted – owe something of their appeal to the fact that they have made their own noteworthy contributions within this general framework of exposition. James's employment of experiences drawn from a wide range of human activity not only served to illuminate the successive stages of his thesis, it also established what a critical admirer once described as the 'anecdotal pattern' of all such studies. Other methods of presentation were bound to emerge in the course of time. James himself warmly welcomed F. W. H. Myers's article on 'The Subliminal Self' as a disclosure of 'an entirely unsuspected peculiarity in the constitution of human nature'. A further disclosure was to appear some years later when another article, this time by a comparatively unknown Viennese doctor, was expanded to become a book under the title *Totem and Taboo* (1913). This startlingly original concatenation of religion, anthropology, the concept of the unconscious and the phenomena of mental derangement, provoked a fiercely hostile reaction. Religion, it was said, which was man's grateful response to God as He had divinely and historically revealed Himself, was being explained away as a chronic mental aberration. This criticism was substantially correct, but it overlooked the possibility that many of the arguments advanced by Freud would in course of time be shown to be capable of positive and creative interpretations.

Despite opposition – or, perhaps, because of it – developments of this radical reassessment of the psychological nature of religion followed with the result that many of the conclusions of the more traditionally minded psychologists were seen to be in need of substantial revision. This need had already been envisaged, not by a psychologist, but by the most eminent of British anthropologists, Sir James Frazer, who several years before, in a notable tribute to the life's work of William Robertson Smith, argued prophetically that the time would come when the religions of the world would no longer be regarded from the angle of their veracity or falsehood, but 'as phenomena of consciousness to be studied like any other aspect of human nature'.[1] Subsequent writers expanded the former somewhat restricted concentration upon the psychology of conversion, morals, asceticism and the more exotic forms of mysticism in the Christianity of the West, to a study of religion as a *universal* phenomenon and a dominant factor in the history of human development. The result has been that today psychological studies of religion borrow substantially from such disciplines as anthropology, comparative religion, the hypotheses of evolution and from the work of the two men whose contributions dominate the whole field of modern psychology – Freud and Jung. This has led to a rapid increase of public interest in religion as a psychological activity and at the same time to a series of specialized studies of religion from the psycho-analytical and analytical points of view. But the variety of these studies is such that no one clear picture of the psychological nature of religion has as yet emerged. None the less certain conclusions have become generally acceptable.

It is now widely agreed that psychology, whether it be defined as a science or not, is not concerned with the uniqueness of any one particular religion (though it is difficult to avoid the conclusion that certain religions convey a higher degree of reality than others) nor yet with the validity of any particular set of beliefs. Psychology is concerned with the reactions of the human psyche, its responses, collective and individual, to that Reality which, in whatever way it be described and experienced, is at one and the same time the source of all religious experience as well as that ultimate satisfaction for which the human soul craves, whether this craving be described as an aspiration for the Divine, a re-orientation of personality and purpose (conversion), the urge to individuation or the quest for some form of mystical union. The one fundamental assumption in contemporary psychologies of religion, however varied their approaches and conclusions, is that there are psychological motivations and responses

[1] *The Gorgon's Head* (1927) pp. 281–2.

which are common to all known forms of religion, whether primitive, highly developed or historical, and that it is with these motivations and their related activities that psychology has to deal.

Religion begins in experience. It is this fact that makes it a proper subject for psychological study. This has now been accepted by many who in earlier decades rejected the possibility that religion could be made the subject of psychological analysis without serious harm. It is now realized that even theological presentations of religious experiences (whatever their creedal or revelationary criteria) proceed from common psychological motivations, from man's natural impulse to record, communicate and interpret experiences that have an all-compelling and unique significance. Metaphysics, as a highly intellectualized activity, is no less psychologically motivated than the lowliest and simplest forms of religious faith and practice since it is the intellectual result of man's instinctual curiosity and his inherent desire for explanation. It is significant that today some of the most stimulating studies in the psychology of religion come from men with established theological loyalties who have not hesitated to use the contributions of the two greatest psychologists of this century (however diametrically opposed their views on religion may be) as the means of elucidating man's responses to the Divine. Modern studies have found the concepts of analytical psychology particularly valuable when dealing with the most representative of all religious responses, namely, prayer, worship and religious experience (whether involuntary or humanly induced). Psychology can of itself offer no opinion as to the ultimate significance of these practices, what it can do is to indicate how these activities are related to the psychical constitution of man when he confronts, or is confronted by, the High and the Holy.

Part I

PSYCHOLOGICAL THEORIES AND RELIGION

Chapter I

PSYCHOLOGY AND RELIGION

The value of studies in the psychology of religion has in recent years been increased greatly by contributions from archaeology, anthropology, ethnology and sociology. But the difficulties of defining the exact boundaries of psychology, and the fact that the nature of religion is such that it eludes exhaustive definition, present us with problems of a special kind.

The Contemporary Position

Recent studies in comparative religion show that all religions – despite considerable diversities of belief and practice – exhibit similarities which need to be explained by something more than processes of assimilation, conventionalization and cultural diffusion, though each of these factors plays an important part.[1] These similarities spring from such facts as the universality of human needs, spiritual no less than physical; from the same impulse towards unity and completeness; and from the same awareness of powers that appear to operate within the world and yet are external to it. Man is a religious animal by birth, culture and inheritance, and as such his religious life can be examined psychologically without any verdict being passed upon the validity of his beliefs and their individual and corporate expression. The validity of spiritual truths is a matter upon which no psychologist *qua* psychologist can pronounce an opinion.[2] It may be true that:

> Religion is a difficult and refractory subject of study . . . It is not easy to dissect with the cold knife of logic what can only be accepted with a

[1] See Appendix III.

[2] In the *Psychopathology of Everyday Life* (1904) Freud gave an early expression of his naturalistic outlook on religion: 'I believe in fact that a great part of the mythological view of the world, which reaches far into the most modern religions, is nothing other than psychological processes projected into the outer world. The obscure apprehending of the psychical factors and relationships of the unconscious is mirrored – it is hard to put it otherwise; one has to use the analogy with

complete surrender of heart. It seems impossible to comprehend with reason that which encompasses mankind with love and supreme wisdom.[1]

None the less the fact that religion is an active element in human life at all levels makes it imperative that we should attempt to estimate its nature and activities in terms of contemporary psychology.

As a discipline, psychology is concerned with body and soul (*psyche*), but it is not restricted to a study of their relationship. It is clear that psychology, while it cannot ignore the physiological aspects of man's nervous system, is neither a biological study nor yet an entirely objective examination of man's instinctual and emotional responses to his environment. If psychology is regarded as a study of the will, it calls not only for some consideration of the 'end' (*telos*) towards which man strives and is attracted, it also invites a philosophical assessment of the values which endow that end with something more than a purely practical nature. Life is never a purely practical affair, otherwise man living at primitive and dangerous levels of existence would never have thought it worth while to blow through a hollow reed in an attempt to make musical sounds which had no 'practical' purpose.

Furthermore, psychology shows that man does not always live on the same level of consciousness. There is the level of ordinary everyday awareness, but this awareness is continually subject to fluctuations of attention, to such common experiences as forgetfulness, daydreaming, fatigue and unexpected intrusions of memories and their emotional associations. But the activities of the psyche are not limited to conscious awareness. Some hours of every twenty-four are passed in sleep, and in sleep man becomes aware of another life which often makes his waking experience seem to be little more than the proscenium of a drama which, for beauty, mystery, strangeness and horror, transcends his daily life, so that he cannot but believe that he has a 'double' that is not limited to the confines of his body. By itself, anthropology cannot explain fully how man came to believe that he has a soul that is independent of his conscious awareness. But psychology, having proved empirically the subliminal activity of the

---

paranoia – in the construction of a *super-sensible reality* which science has to retranslate into the psychology of the unconscious. One could venture in this manner to resolve the myths of Paradise, the Fall of Man, of God, of Good and Evil, of Immortality, and so on, thus transforming Metaphysics into Metapsychology.' Quoted with comment in Ernest Jones: *Sigmund Freud* (1957) Vol. III. pp. 377–8.

[1] Bronislaw Malinowski: *The Foundations of Faith and Morals* (1934–1935).

psyche, is able to offer explanations of how primitive man, as a result of his experiences with dreams and the phenomena of death, came to formulate some concept of a 'double' (soul) which was connected with the differential between a body that breathes and a body that has ceased to breathe. A living example of breath thought of as soul is given by Jung from his own researches among the mountain tribesmen of the Elgonyi who, in the morning at the rising of the sun, 'hold their hands before their mouths and spit or blow into them vigorously. Then they turn their hands round and hold the palms forward to the sun.' Jung makes this comment on this particular ceremony:

> it is an offering to the sun which for these natives is *mungu* – that is *mana* or divine – only at the moment of rising. If they have spittle on their hands, this is the substance which, according to primitive belief, contains the personal *mana*, the force that cures, conjures and sustains life. If they breathe upon their hands, breath is wind and spirit. . . . The action means 'I offer my living spirit to God'. It is a wordless, acted prayer, which could equally well be spoken: 'Lord, into thy hands, I commend my spirit.' [1]

This connexion remains to this day in Christian thought where the Holy Spirit is referred to in terms of 'the wind bloweth where it listeth and thou hearest the sound thereof . . . so is everyone that is born of the spirit'.[2]

The soul was also connected with other aspects of the body, such as blood, the heart, shadow or sometimes the 'name', but of all these tropes, blood and breath[3] were those most frequently associated with the soul. Blood, like breath, is one of the most natural symbols of life. This explains why blood plays such a prominent part in sacrifices (as we shall see later); it is one of the most significant means by which

[1] Jung: *Modern Man in Search of a Soul* (1936) pp. 172 ff.

[2] John iii. 8.

[3] Among the numerous terms used for *breath* there are many which are linguistically related to terms which refer to *soul* or *psyche*. For instance:

Akkadian and Assyrian:	*napištu*	= breath, life, soul.
Hebrew:	*nephesh*	= breath, life, soul or person.
Arabic:	*tanaffus*	= to fetch a deep breath.
	nafs	= breath of life.
Greek:	*psyche*	= breath or soul.
Stoic:	*pneuma*	= breath or spirit.
Latin:	*anima* & *animus*	= from Greek, *anemos* = soul and wind.
Sanskrit:	*ātman* & *prāna*	= breath, wind or soul.

man is able to make 'a lively sacrifice'. Hence the expression 'the blood of the Lamb' who, in Christian theology, 'taketh away the sins of the world'.[1]

A study of the beliefs of primitive peoples[2] shows that in many of them, man regarded the soul not only as a 'double' but in many cases believed in a plurality of souls, each being identified with some function of the body. The Keokuk Indians, for instance, distinguished between the soul of the heart, the soul of the flesh, of life, name and family; while the Melanesians believed that a man could have as many as seven souls. In the West these functional aspects of the soul were identified with the faculties of the unified psyche. But in addition to this variety of psychical functions, it is clear that in most religions and at all levels of culture, the soul (psyche) was believed to be *the* means whereby man apprehended the all-surrounding, all-pervading Mystery of life.[3]

Whatever other aspects the psychology of religion may have to deal with, for our present purpose it is the study of how the soul of man, both consciously and unconsciously, responds to the mystery of life and death, and to the impingement of an environment which in many ways appears to be even more mysteriously alive than man himself. But if this is the main concern of our study, we have yet to define what is meant by the term 'religion'.

Definitions

Religion includes not only the beliefs, customs, traditions and rites which belong to particular social groupings, it also involves individual experiences. Any definition which stresses the communal aspects of religion to the exclusion of the individual's psychic life, is defective since it is the individual's apprehension of some supreme Object, Power or Principle that constitutes one of the most important features of religion.

Religion embraces such a wide variety of data that it is not surprising that Professor C. C. J. Webb should have said: 'I do not

[1] John i. 29, and Rev. v. 6.
[2] See Appendix I.
[3] The ancient Hebrews were forbidden to eat flesh unless the blood (the soul) had first been drained from it. 'I will set my face against the [man] that eateth blood, and will cut him off from among his people. For the life of the flesh is in the blood; and I have given it to you upon the altar to make atonement for your souls; for it is the blood that maketh atonement by reason of the life.' Lev. xvii. 10, 11; see also: Deut. xii. 16, and 1 Sam. xiv. 32, 33.

believe that Religion *can* be defined.' [1] Other writers, however, have made noteworthy attempts at definition. Sir James Frazer said that by religion

> I understand a propitiation or conciliation of powers superior to man which are believed to direct and control the course of nature and of human life. Thus defined, religion consists of two elements, a theoretical and a practical, namely a belief in powers higher than man and an attempt to propitiate or please them.

To this definition, Frazer added the useful comment that 'belief clearly comes first, since we must believe in the existence of a divine being before we can attempt to please him. But unless the belief leads to a corresponding practice, it is not a religion but merely a theology.' [2] A different emphasis is to be found in Émile Durkheim's definition, where the emphasis is on belief and practice within a social community:

> A religion is a unified system of beliefs and practices relative to sacred things, that is to say, things set apart and forbidden – beliefs and practices which unite into one single moral community called a Church, all those who adhere to them. The second element which thus finds a place in our definition is no less essential than the first; for by showing that the idea of religion is inseparable from that of the Church, it makes it clear that religion should be an eminently collective thing.[3]

To this definition, Durkheim adds, in a footnote, that in an earlier definition he had defined religious beliefs exclusively by their obligatory character, but that he proposed to amend this definition by showing that their obligatoriness was the result of their being imposed by the group upon its members.

On the other hand, a definition by Professor George Galloway placed the main emphasis upon the individual and his psychological needs. Religion is that which refers to 'Man's faith in a power beyond himself whereby he seeks to satisfy emotional needs and gain stability of life, and which he expresses in acts of worship and service'.[4] To which definition, Galloway adds that

> The cognitive side of the religious consciousness is represented by faith, and faith is stimulated by emotion and posits the object which will satisfy the needs of the inner life. One of the most urgent and constant of

[1] See C. C. J. Webb: *Group Theories of Religion* (1916).
[2] James Frazer: *The Golden Bough*: abridged edition (1925) p. 50.
[3] E. Durkheim: *The Elementary Forms of the Religious Life* (1954) p. 47.
[4] G. Galloway: *The Philosophy of Religion* (1914) p. 184.

> man's needs is that which is expressed in the desire for self-conservation, or, as we have put it, for stability of life in the face of the manifold forces which threaten and limit him. The practical aspect is denoted by the acts of worship and service which belong to the nature of religion.[1]

The last sentence of this definition will occupy our attention in the second part of this book.

Two of the most useful definitions yet provided by any writers on the psychology of religion are to be found in J. Bissett Pratt's well-known *The Religious Consciousness* and in R. H. Thouless's much-quoted *Introduction to the Psychology of Religion.*

> Religion is the serious and social attitude of individuals or communities toward the power or powers which they conceive as having ultimate control over their interests and destinies. . . . This definition has . . . one or two characteristics to which I wish to call the reader's attention. First, it defines religion as an 'attitude.' . . . The word 'attitude' shall here be used to cover that *responsive* side of consciousness which is found in such things as attention, interest, expectancy, feeling, tendencies to action etc. . . . The advantages of defining religion as an attitude are sufficiently manifest. It shows that religion is not a matter of any one 'department' of psychic life but involves the whole man. It includes what there was of truth in the historical attempts to identify religion with feeling, belief or will. And it draws attention to the fact that religion is immediately subjective, thus differing from science (which emphasizes 'content' rather than 'attitude'); and yet it points to the other fact also that religion involves and presupposes the acceptance of the objective. Religion is the attitude of a self towards an object in which the self genuinely believes.[2]

Dr R. H. Thouless, having considered various definitions by other writers, came to the conclusion that any definition of religion to be adequate must include at least three factors:

> a mode of behaviour, a system of intellectual beliefs and a system of feelings. In order to find a complete and satisfactory definition, we must further enquire what is the particular mark of the conduct, beliefs and feelings in question which characterises them as religious. . . . Our definition will then run in some such form as this: *Religion is a felt practical relationship with what is believed in as a superhuman being or beings.*[3]

To this definition, Dr Thouless adds that

> there are two terms in common use in the psychology of religion which must be explained. These are the *religious consciousness*, and *religious*

[1] G. Galloway: *The Philosophy of Religion* (1914) p. 184.
[2] J. B. Pratt: *The Religious Consciousness* (1930) pp. 2–3.
[3] R. H. Thouless: *An Introduction to the Psychology of Religion* (1936) pp. 3–4.

> *experience*. The religious consciousness is that part of religion which is present to the mind and is open to examination by introspection. It is the mental side of religious activity. *Religious experience* is a vaguer term used to describe the feeling element in the religious consciousness – the feelings which lead to religious belief or are the effects of religious behaviour.[1] . . . The main business of the psychology of religion is to study the religious consciousness. But it is impossible to study that alone; we must investigate religious behaviour as well.[2]

These definitions together with their psychological explanations are, however, not entirely representative of all the definitions that have been made in the course of many years. In fact so many attempts have been made to arrive at a satisfactory definition that Leuba was able to select forty-eight definitions, to which he added two of his own, for inclusion in his famous *Psychological Study of Religion* (1912). An analysis of these definitions of religion, together with those written subsequently, reveals that what is there defined is not in all cases the same 'activity', for the term 'religion' like the word 'God' is one of those 'umbrella' words which gathers under its protection implications and meanings some of which are plainly opposed to or corrective of others.

Leuba divided his rich collection of definitions into two groups, those which treat religion as 'the recognition of a mystery pressing for interpretation', and those which adopt Schleiermacher's view that religion is 'a feeling of absolute dependence upon God'. To these two schools of thought, Leuba added yet a third. Religion is 'the *propitiation* or *conciliation* of powers which are believed to direct and control the course of nature and human life'.[3] (A definition which is substantially the same as that advanced by Pratt.) To which we must add – since no psychology of religion can possibly be written that does not

[1] One school of modern psychological study – the Behaviourist – adopts the wholly unsatisfactory attitude that psychology is concerned with *the study of behaviour only*. It repudiates all study of the mind as being a non-experimental concept. For this reason it is not possible to accept any Behaviourist verdict on religion. Whatever religion involves, it clearly involves a consideration of how man's mind reacts to and formulates explanations of the content of experience and its environment. Religion includes at least three factors, belief, feeling and behaviour (which includes things-done and things-not-to-be-done, ritual and taboo), no single one of which can operate by itself.

[2] op. cit. p. 5.

[3] The fact that the Buddha in his opposition to Hindu metaphysics did not share this belief in various deities nor that worship should be made to them, must not obscure the fact that later forms of Buddhism, e.g. Mahāyāna Buddhism in particular, do in actual practice show that they have restored this belief in the existence of supernatural powers to whom worship must be offered.

quite early on begin to quote from William James – the comment that because there are so many definitions of religion and the fact that they are

> so different from one another is enough to prove that the word 'religion' can not stand for any single principle or essence. . . . The theorizing mind tends always to the over-simplification of its materials. . . . In the broadest and most general terms possible, one might say that religious life consists in the belief that there is an unseen order, and that our supreme good lies in harmoniously adjusting ourselves thereto. This belief and this adjustment are the religious attitude of the soul. . . . Moreover, there must be something solemn, serious and tender about any attitude which we denominate religious.[1]

It seems clear, therefore, that no one particular attitude to religion will suffice. Intellect, behaviour involving the operation both of will and feeling (as well as of other factors which we have not yet mentioned) are all involved. But what is not clear is the way in which these elements are related to and what is their specific importance in religion, since they all are involved in every discipline (sacred and secular) that engages human effort.

Leuba himself emphasized the importance of the will as the operative factor in religion viewed as behaviour, but wisely added that he did not exclude from his own concept of religion aspects which do not express themselves in overt acts, in rites of propitiation, submission or adoration. *Active* religion includes certain kinds of behaviour proceeding from the operation of the will and, as we shall see, from instinctual dispositions, while *passive* religion is that form in which the feeling-attitude is more prominent and where the psyche is acted upon by, rather than acts towards, the Object of its devotion. Archbishop Söderblom argued that the essential element in religion is neither formal belief nor organized worship but a response to the 'tabu-holy'.[2] The psychology of religion must, therefore, include the study of man's response to that power which he regards as 'sacred'.[3]

[1] William James: *Varieties of Religious Experience*: 36th edn (1928) pp. 26 ff.

[2] N. Söderblom: *Das Werden des Gottesglauben* (1916) p. 211.

[3] 'At bottom, the only helpful thing one can say of the sacred in general is contained in the very definition of the term: that it is the opposite of profane. As soon as one attempts to give a clear statement of the nature, the *modality* of that opposition, one strikes difficulty. No formula, however elementary, will cover the labyrinthine complexity of the facts.' Roger Caillois: *L'Homme et le sacré*: quoted by Mircea Eliade: *Patterns in Comparative Religion* (1958) p. xii. To which Professor Eliade adds that among the facts of this labyrinthine complexity he himself includes taboo, ritual, symbol, myth, demon, god – 'but it would be an outrageous simplification to make such a list tell the whole story'.

Before we can proceed further we must attempt to see what anthropology has to say about religion and culture at early levels of human development.

Anthropology and Early Cultures

Anthropology and ethnology show that the institutions and customs of man at comparatively low levels of development exhibit a striking similarity in widely separated parts of the world; the relics of every prehistoric society so far discovered show that all peoples knew how to make fire; that wrought flints of the Palaeolithic and Neolithic types have been found in all parts of the world and that artefacts[1] presumed to have religious associations existed at all levels of prehistoric civilizations. Such evidence may be taken to imply that early man shared 'in an ultimately identical tradition'.[2] The existence of such a tradition is attested by what Professor Herbert Kühn has to say at the conclusion of his study of the prehistoric art of the Pyrenees:

> From out of the caverns hidden deep in the recesses of the earth, mysterious things have appeared. Caves have found voices and speak to us about men of long ago, men far off from us and yet so near. Men, very like ourselves. Their hopes were comparable with ours, their wishes and their dreams not so very different from our own. What spurred on prehistoric men, what set their tasks, what provided their goal was what we may call the complex of birth and death. . . . Standing, as it were, on the surface of to-day, we can look down into the profound pit of our remote past, and, there, as in a mirror, see ourselves . . . beings like ourselves. We see Man struggling for existence, fighting with the mighty Powers to which he is subservient. . . . From out of this arduous and ardent food-quest arose the great spiritual qualities which have served and still serve us as aid, protection and encouragement in our struggle for existence. First of all religion expressed in magic, wizardry, ritual dances, ceremonial garments, enchantment, sacred song . . . and Art, close linked with religion, then as in later epochs. Next sustained and coherent thought, subjective concepts, magic, experience of strange phenomena; a magical conception of the universe. Lastly, we have philosophy. All three realms of the spiritual life, religion, art and philosophy, have their beginnings in that world of prehistoric Man.[3]

---

[1] 'The "bullroarer" is found always as a sacred instrument employed in religious mysteries, in New Mexico, in Australia, in New Zealand, in ancient Greece and in Africa: while it is a peasant boy's plaything in England.' Andrew Lang: *Custom and Myth* (1904) p. 31.

[2] L. R. Farnell: *The Evolution of Religion* (1905) p. 9.

[3] Herbert Kühn: *On the Track of Prehistoric Man* (1958) pp. 184–5.

It seems reasonable, therefore, to suppose that the cultural similarities found at early levels of society are related to basic psychological similarities; for in much the same way as the physical body is essentially the same everywhere – whatever the pigmentation – so the mind of man everywhere exhibits certain basic characteristics. Such widespread customs as Exogamy, Endogamy, and Totemism, would seem to originate from much the same mental reactions to life and environment.

> If we look back upon the history of thought, it is obvious that there was once a time when the amount of divergence must have been exceedingly small . . . we see in primitive and rudimentary societies that a certain oneness of all thought is characteristic of the lower levels.[1]

But we must set against this argument the theory of cultural diffusion. This theory, less popular today than when it was energetically propagated by Grafton Elliot Smith and W. J. Perry, must be briefly referred to here because, if it were true universally, it would have an important bearing upon the validity of Jung's argument for the existence of the collective unconscious (objective psyche). Elliot Smith and W. J. Perry argued that the origins of civilization were traceable to the genius of pre-Dynastic Egypt; that the similarities between different civilizations in different parts of the world were due to cultural diffusion; that migration and travel were the means whereby the beliefs and practices of one civilization were carried into distant parts of the world. An impressive amount of evidence for inter-continental travel has been adduced in recent years by some highly adventurous expeditions which have shown that contact between widely separated continents and islands was possible in early times.[2] But allowing for such transmissions and migrations, it still remains necessary, as R. R. Marett more than once pointed out, to consider the psychological aspects of cultural transmission. If some men in one part of the world borrow ideas and practices from another civilization, while other peoples decline to do so, the explanation is to be found in the psychological motives involved and the level of social development attained. Because man everywhere appears to possess a psychology that is basically the same he is able

[1] Stanley A. Cook: *The Study of Religions* (1914) p. 84.

[2] Thor Heyerdahl: *Kon-Tiki* (1950). Professor Gordon Childe has pointed out that the Polynesians of Oceania, using stone tools, were able to build boats over one hundred feet long, capable of carrying a hundred persons with provisions for a voyage of over a thousand miles. See Gordon Childe: *What Happened in History* (1942) pp. 75 ff.

to assimilate customs and practices which he imagines will promote his well-being, and to reject those which he thinks will imperil it. Furthermore, it is difficult to believe, more so now than when this theory was first advanced, that the only inventive minds were those of pre-Dynastic Egypt. Archaeological discoveries in various parts of the world do not support Elliot Smith's theory.[1]

It seems more reasonable to assume that Palaeolithic culture which once covered more than half the world was associated with a corresponding type of mind,[2] and that all the races which passed through this cultural stage had a common psychology. This argument is closely associated with yet another modern theory – evolution. Since the evolutionary development of the brain seems to be related to the development of beliefs and customs among primitive peoples we must pause to ask what is meant by 'primitive man' and what do we know of his psychological development?

Primitive Man and Religion

The word 'primitive' is usually taken to mean that which is near to an 'original' state, but when this term is applied to man it refers to the stage at which man becomes clearly distinguishable from his animal ancestry. Fossilized remains of early man show that while his physical frame was closely related to that of anthropoid apes, his cranial structure and capacity exhibited significant differences. The chief difference seems to be connected with the evolutionary development of the pre-frontal regions of the brain. A study of the physical development of the human skull shows that those areas which are associated with imagination were well developed in early man, but that those areas of the primitive cortex which are associated with rational control and co-ordination were deficient. This physiological fact in itself furnishes one criterion by which to distinguish between 'primitive' and 'modern' man.

[1] See for instance: Sir John Marshall: *Mohenjo-Daro and the Indus Civilization* (1931), where it is shown that the most ancient of the cities uncovered at Harappa and Mohenjo-Daro have cultural connexions with Mesopotamia and Susiana. See also: E. Mackay: *The Indus Civilization* (1935); Stuart Piggott: *Prehistoric India* (1950); Sir Mortimer Wheeler: *Early India and Pakistan* (1959); and W. F. Albright: *From the Stone Age to Christianity* (revised edn. 1957).

[2] Arnold Toynbee has a well-documented presentation of what he calls 'The Uniformity Theory and the Diffusion Theory' in Annex I.C (iii) b, of Vol. I. *A Study of History* (1934) pp. 424–40, in which he says 'the diffusion of the antecedent civilization may provide the stimulus to creation, but it cannot itself be identical with the creative force, since, *ex hypothesi*, it emanates from a soul which has already become impotent'.

If we study the mentality of people whose cranial development may be described as 'primitive' we see that primitive minds had difficulty in distinguishing clearly between animate and inanimate objects, with the result that many of their concepts appear to have been vague and fluctuating. (The relevance of this for such concepts as those of animatism and animism needs no special emphasis.) As the pre-frontal areas of the brain developed, man became more and more 'eye-minded'. This follows the general course of physical evolution in which, as the olfactory areas of vertebrates decrease, an increase is observed in those regions of the brain which are concerned with visual imagery and audible impressions. This development is of some importance for the religion of primitive man. The fact that all religions exhibit the presence of powerful imagery may in part be due to man's 'eye-mindedness'. This tendency to 'think' in pictures continues to operate strongly whenever man is confronted with aspects of experience with which his intellectual processes find it difficult to deal. Children between the ages of three and six embody their experiences in characters whose activities express pictorially the child's non-intellectual account of the world about and within him. The psychological development of children bears a very close resemblance to that of the primitive mind and this fact is of great importance for the psychology of religion. As his brain developed, man became endowed with powers of co-ordination and finally with the power of speech, a development which represents one of the great 'crises' in human history. It meant that the multiple pictures expressive of primitive experience were brought to a brilliant focus – the 'word'. Multiple mental pictures became a single word but such words retained these pre-linguistic pictorial associations.[1] Paintings of the Aurignacian and Magdalenian ages on the walls of deep caves in the Dordogne show not only the highly pictorial nature of early thinking, but also a feature which explains the rituals of primitive religion no less than those of later times. These pictures, painted in places where it would have been physically impossible to take living models, show the same obsessive preoccupation with exact detail as distinguished the performances of religious rites where a single mistake or omission was held to impair the efficacy of the whole cere-

[1] The language of primitive peoples is markedly pictorial, lacking the power to embody in purely intellectual terms ideas expressive of class and species. The Tasmanians, for example, possessed all sorts of words with which to refer to different kinds of trees but they had no general term for 'tree'. Jung refers to this kind of thinking as 'concretism': see *Psychological Types* (1938) p. 533.

monial. This was equally true of rites performed in late Roman times.[1] This preoccupation with correctness of detail arises from that element of fear which played such an influential part in the religion of primitive man and which continues to do so in many of the religions and superstitions of modern times.[2] These are matters which we shall discuss more fully in subsequent chapters.

[1] The efficacy of such rites was believed to be directly dependent upon the use of the *appropriate name* of the god whose aid was required. The functional aid of a 'special' god could be secured in some particular set of circumstances only by using his *real* name. Hence many names were employed as invocatory alternatives in order to avoid missing the essential name of the god whose help was desired. In classical religions (and also in Christian rituals) 'the art of right address became a sacerdotal technique' the efficacy of which depended upon exact and flawless repetition. See G. Wissowa: *Religion und Kultus der Römer* (1912) Vol. 2. p. 37.

[2] See Oskar Pfister: *Some Applications of Psycho-analysis* (1923) pp. 330 ff.

Chapter II

THE HISTORY OF THE PSYCHOLOGY OF RELIGION

We may assume that man from very early times was able to reflect in some way upon his own awareness of life, but there is no record of these reflections until quite late in human history. For our purpose we propose to see how certain men in the later periods of Western thought approached the subject of human consciousness, selecting only those views which eventually resolved themselves into the psychology of religion.

Plato and Aristotle

Greek interest in the soul (psyche) was a natural development of a general philosophical interest in the natuie and origin of the cosmos. Zeno's conception of the world as pervaded by a universal principle of life (hylozoism) was an extension of man's projection of his own self-consciousness on to the phenomenal world. This interest in a world closely related to and yet distinct from man, served to emphasize the psychological distinction between the objective world and the mind which contemplates it. It soon became apparent that knowledge depended upon something other than sensory experience; that the human senses needed to be corrected by reason and reflection. But if our senses can sometimes deceive us, what grounds have we for placing greater reliance upon reason? Furthermore, since knowledge includes personal factors how can we distinguish between what is called objective and subjective?

It was not until the time of Socrates (469–399 B.C.), Plato (429–347 B.C.), and Aristotle (384–322 B.C.) that we find a consistent attempt to formulate a theory of knowledge and to arrive at a psychological estimate of the nature of man. Socrates, according to Plato, introduced a virtual revolution into Greek philosophy by concentrating (in contradistinction to the Ionian philosophers who were chiefly concerned with the external world) upon man's *inner* nature. But it was Plato's presentation of the theory of knowledge which provided, through the mouth of Socrates, a psychological distinction of fundamental importance. Knowledge, for Plato, differs essentially from opinions based on sensory experience. Knowledge arises from what Plato called 'Ideas'. These ideas are not derived from sensory phenomena, they exist independently of the world of space and time. By treating Ideas as objective 'universals' Plato had to show how man becomes aware of their existence. To do this he had to explain that man has a soul (psyche) which resides temporarily in the body. In the interludes between one incarnation and the next, the soul in the heavenly places is able to contemplate these eternal Ideas. When the soul again becomes resident in a physical body, it sometimes finds itself involved in situations which remind it of the Ideas which it had known during its residence in the 'heavenlies'. It is these 'reminiscences' which are the basis of all real knowledge.

Aristotle rejected Plato's explanation, saying that knowledge began in down-to-earth experience; that it was based upon experience of individual things (Plato's 'particulars') which were not to be treated as imperfect copies of universals laid up in heaven. The soul, as intelligence, is able to classify particulars in general terms, and these general terms exist as mental but not immortal concepts.

The psychological relevance of Plato's and Aristotle's views is not restricted to their rival theories of knowledge. We find in Plato the first adumbration of a concept which we today know as the 'unconscious'. Socrates asks 'whether it is possible to know the same thing both sharply and dully, to know close at hand but not at a distance, to know violently and gently . . . and countless other questions',[1] which seems to indicate that Plato was making a distinction between 'focal' and 'marginal' attention. Socrates proceeds to ask whether it is possible to have experiences and not be aware of them, and what part memory plays in such a process?

> Do you suppose that you could get anybody to admit that the memory a man has of past feelings he no longer feels is anything like the feeling at the time when he is feeling it? Far from it. Or, that he would refuse to admit that it is possible for one and the same person to know and not to know the one and the same thing?[2]

For Socrates man is the subject of impressions not all of which remain on the stage of conscious awareness. Plato does not discuss

[1] *Theaetetus*: 165 B. [2] op. cit. 166 B.

why some impressions can be recalled and others cannot, but we find Socrates in the *Republic*, when discussing the nature of dreams, referring to desires

> which bestir themselves when the gentler part of the soul slumbers and the control of reason is withdrawn; then the wild-beast in us, full-fed with meat and drink, becomes rampant in us . . . it will cast away all shame and prudence and at such moments will stick at nothing. In phantasy it will not shrink from intercourse with a mother or anyone else, man, god or brute, or from forbidden food or any deed of blood. . . .[1]

Here we seem to have a clear anticipation of the dynamic nature of the unconscious.

Much the same matter is discussed by Aristotle for whom memory is dependent upon the retention of images. Aristotle envisages these images continuing in such a form that when they are not present in normal states of awareness, they none the less exist potentially: 'sensation is either a faculty like sight or an activity, like seeing. But we may have an image even when neither the one nor the other is present; for example, the images in dreams.' [2] Aristotle points out that in addition to seeing and hearing, *we can be aware* that we see and hear. '. . . the mind has some ingredient in its composition which makes it the object of thought. The mind itself is included among the objects which can be thought.' [3] This is virtually the position which Plotinus developed five centuries later. The soul in knowing itself 'knows that there is something better than itself' [4] and, says Plotinus, we can no more doubt these higher experiences than we can doubt our actual existence.

With the exception of Plotinus there is, subsequent to Aristotle, little of psychological interest until we come to St Augustine of Hippo (A.D. 353–430).

Augustine of Hippo

Augustine insisted that the inner life of man is *sui generis* and that introspection is the method by which it can be studied. He arrived at these conclusions by means of the neo-Platonic doctrine that the soul pervades the body, that it is immortal because it contains imperishable Ideas and is the basis of all mental activities. Augustine made

[1] *The Republic*: IX. 571: Trans. F. M. Cornford.
[2] *De Anima*: Bk III. chap. iii. 7.
[3] op. cit. Bk III. chap. iv. 10, 11.
[4] Ennead V. Bk VIII. 4.

yet another notable contribution to psychology, saying that it is not possible to doubt one's own living experience, a position which he set out in his *Soliloquia*: 'thought and, therefore, the existence of the thinker are the most certain of all things',[1] and again:

> when we reflect upon ourselves, we find in ourselves not only sensations, but also an internal sense (*sensus interior*) which makes of the former its objects (for we have knowledge of our sensations but the external senses are unable to perceive their own sensations) and, finally reason, which knows both the interior sense and itself.

Augustine associated this *sensus interior* with the means whereby man could arrive at a knowledge of God.

> That which judges is always superior to that which is judged; but that, according to which judgements are rendered, is also superior to that which judges. The human reason perceives that there is something higher than itself; for it is changeable, now knowing, now not knowing, now seeking after knowledge, now not, now correctly, now incorrectly judging: but truth itself, which is the norm according to which it judges, must be unchangeable . . . hence it is impossible to doubt the existence of truth itself. Now the unchangeable truth is God . . . All ideas are in God. He is the eternal ground of all form, who imparted to created objects their temporal forms.[2]

This *sensus interior* finds a prominent place in the carefully systematized psychology of Avicenna (A.D. 980–1037), a system which is substantial evidence of the high level of Muslim culture at this time. Avicenna followed Aristotle's lead by asserting that the soul is the intelligence which informs the body of man, giving him the power to make concepts from the multiplicity of sensory objects by which he is surrounded. Mind, for Avicenna, is manifest in three ascending forms, vegetable, animal and human, but only the human mind possesses intelligence. The Muslim world by Avicenna's time had worked out a general theory of consciousness and had already found the need for some such concept as that of the unconscious, but several centuries had to elapse before the full significance of such a concept emerged.

Scholasticism

The thought of the Middle Ages begins with John Scotus Erigena (fl. A.D. 850) who believed that faith and reason were manifestations

[1] op. cit. II. 1.
[2] *De Lib. Arb.* II. 3 et seq.: quoted Ueberweg: *History of Philosophy* (1875) Vol. I. pp. 339–40.

of the same divine principle. This connexion reappears in Anselm of Bec (A.D. 1034–1109). Its psychological interest is that faith, which for Anselm is the condition for understanding Christian truth (*fides praecedens intellectum*), is a condition achieved by the interaction of emotion and the will. It is important to note that Anselm meant by *fides* not only truth derived from Scripture and the dogmas of the Church but also something that is derived from the believer's own religious experiences, a point of great importance for the psychology of religion.

The Schoolmen of the earlier Middle Ages were strongly influenced by neo-Platonic thought and assumed, as had Augustine, that man could study his own inner life, an assumption which contributed not a little to the attempts of medieval mystics to record their own psychological experiences. The influence of Aristotelian thought in the second half of the Middle Ages is seen most brilliantly in the works of St Thomas Aquinas (A.D. 1224–1275) who, by adopting Aristotle's views about man's faculties being dependent upon the nature of the soul, was able to avoid Plato's dualism of body and soul. But Aquinas qualified the Aristotelian point of view by saying that the soul as 'form' is a spiritual principle created by God for man's eternal happiness. Man is the microcosm which unites the two realms of matter and form.

In marked contrast to the Thomist views were those of Duns Scotus (A.D. 1264–1308), a Franciscan, who insisted that the will and not the intellect is the most important faculty, thus anticipating by many centuries McDougall's 'hormic' psychology. Like some modern psychologists, Duns Scotus doubted whether 'introspection' could reveal the true nature of man 'since we cannot dig up the roots of our own being'. William of Occam (d. 1349), another Franciscan, made a contribution which appears in later Western thought as the argument that man's soul is endowed with a special faculty by which it is able to apprehend super-sensuous truths. This suggestion arises from the distinction which Occam made between man as limited by the sensory world and man endowed with the 'privilege' of faith. The modernity of Occam's outlook, which is somewhat obscured by medieval terminology, is shown in his three basic assumptions: the value of an appeal to empirical experience; the reality of individual personality; and the fact that the study of personality is a study of objective fact.

It is of interest to note that a man with a very different nature and outlook, the German mystic Meister Eckhart (1260–1327), held that the realities of the soul were more vividly revealed by reflection upon mystical experience than by rational introspections of intellect and will. There is, said Eckhart, 'something in the soul that is uncreated and uncreatable' through which a divine re-birth takes place in the soul of man. This insistence by many medieval thinkers upon the importance of individual experience in religion, and the necessity of spiritual re-birth, assumes new forms as we shall see later when dealing with religious experience and Jung's concept of Individuation.

In the next two centuries there are no developments of major importance except that, during the Reformation, Protestant theologians strongly emphasized the subjective aspects of religion. The more important developments of psychological thought are not seen until the seventeenth century.

The Seventeenth and Eighteenth Centuries

In its reaction to medieval thought, the seventeenth century emphasized the part played by reason but failed to attach sufficient importance to the part played by feeling. Its chief contributions to psychology were made by three of the world's greatest philosophers, Descartes, Locke and Leibniz. Descartes (1596–1650), by insisting that mind and body are totally disparate 'substances', initiated a new debate in the West. He was concerned to give an account of the nature and contents of consciousness as the basis of all knowledge. The mind, according to Descartes, was 'a thinking thing' from which it was but a single step to the position that the mind is that which thinks always. Opposed to Descartes was the English empiricist, John Locke (1632–1704), who held that the mind does not think all the time since the mind could have ideas only when the subject himself was conscious of such mental activity. Locke's criticism of the Cartesian position provided Leibniz (1646–1716) with the opportunity to make his particular contribution. Leibniz agreed with Descartes that the mind thinks all the time, that it contains innate ideas, the existence of which Locke, with his description of the mind as being initially a *tabula rasa*, had denied. If the mind thinks all the time then there must be some ideas which at times lack consciousness. 'I maintain that something goes on in the soul which corresponds to the circulation of the blood, of which we are never conscious, just as those who live near a mill do not perceive the noise it makes.' [1]

[1] Leibniz: *New Essay* p. 47.

Leibniz had, therefore, to explain why some ideas are not in consciousness. He found the explanation in two things, one, a 'lack of attention', and the other in the suggestion that *some impressions are so small* as to elude consciousness. The 'intensity' of these *petites perceptions* is too low to affect consciousness, but awareness, for Leibniz, is built up on perceptions too small to be perceived by themselves – a highly important contribution to modern psychology.

In the next century the concept of the unconscious received a somewhat different treatment from Kant (1724–1804) who, like Leibniz, held that there are 'percepts which we have without being aware of them'. Leibniz believed that the 'unconscious' consisted of multitudinous *petites perceptions*; Kant held that it consisted of *non-conscious processes.* According to Kant there are some mental processes which are not perceptible, their existence is revealed by their knitting together into experiential 'wholes' the material which comes to us through perception and sensation; it is these processes which Kant called the 'blind' functions of the soul.

The Nineteenth Century

In the first half of the nineteenth century, Schopenhauer (1788–1860) gave a much more exact definition of the concept of the unconscious than had any of his predecessors because he was concerned to find a convincing reason why some ideas are remembered and others forgotten. Schopenhauer's explanation was based on the belief that all human activities are directed by the will which is responsible for the emergence and the disappearance of ideas into and out of consciousness. A somewhat similar explanation was offered by Herbart (1776–1841) who suggested that some ideas are forced out of consciousness by other and opposing ideas. Both of these explanations resemble those offered by psycho-analysis, but whereas Schopenhauer and Herbart stressed the importance of conative and intellectual factors, later explanations have emphasized the importance of affective elements.

It is not necessary to refer to Fechner, Hamilton, Reid or Dugald Stewart; it will be sufficient if we consider Carl Gustav Carus whose *Psyche* was published in 1848, and von Hartmann whose *Philosophy of the Unconscious* appeared in 1868 (English translation 1931). Carus, who had been Court Physician to the King of Saxony and was a man of considerable versatility, put forward views about the nature of the unconscious (*Unberwusst*) explaining that the only way to understand man's conscious life was by referring to the unconscious. It is the unconscious aspect of the psyche which is the real subject-matter of psychology – consciousness being nothing more than an instrument for unconscious activities. Much that is later to be found in Jung's theories of the unconscious and of archetypes is anticipated by Carus's exposition, particularly his emphasis upon the non-individualistic nature of the unconscious and its ceaseless activities. It is interesting to note, in view of Jung's statement that God (i.e. the God-imago) is a 'function' of the unconscious, that Carus actually describes the unconscious as 'the creative activity of the Divine'.

Von Hartmann's conception of the unconscious bears a close resemblance to that outlined by Schopenhauer, but he so extended its activities that the unconscious appeared to govern everything in the organic world.[1] The unconscious was distinguished by conative and cognitive activities, but affective impulses were accorded no place of their own, since von Hartmann held that emotion was capable of being resolved into will and thought.

> Will and idea in the unconscious are essential to each other. . . . Whether the will is conscious or not depends on whether the ideas presented to it are or are not conscious. The cognitive aspects of the unconscious are, therefore, quite as important as the conative, and the balance between these is carefully preserved throughout the entire exposition of the subject.[2]

Von Hartmann's views so clearly foreshadow modern psycho-analytic theories that Professor J. C. Flügel comments that 'Freud's work may perhaps be looked upon as a scientification of von Hartmann's philosophy of the unconscious'.[3]

Wundt (1832–1921), whose views also resemble Schopenhauer's, emphasized the part which the emotions and the intellect play in relation to the will which operates both consciously and unconsciously in a purposive manner.[4] Wundt, like Herbart before him, distinguished between marginal and focal attention and between two fields of consciousness, that of general awareness and a more restricted area of focal awareness. These distinctions had been anticipated by F. W. H. Myers (1843–1901) who as a founder member of the Society for Psychical Research contributed a paper to

[1] Cf. C. Spearman: *Psychology Down the Ages* (1937) Vol. I. p. 375.

[2] Quoted by W. L. Northridge: *Modern Theories of the Unconscious* (1924) p. 18.

[3] J. C. Flügel: *A Hundred Years of Psychology* (1933) p. 292.

[4] A view which figures prominently in Francis Aveling's *Personality and Will* (1931).

the Society's *Proceedings* for 1886 on 'The Subliminal Self'. Myers's views may be succinctly summed up in two brief quotations: 'I conceive that no self of which we can here have cognisance is in reality more than a fragment of a larger self revealed in a fashion at once shifting and limited through an organism not so framed as to afford it full satisfaction.' Beneath the level of ordinary awareness, there is a *subliminal* or *ultra-marginal* consciousness whose activities are such that Myers concluded that there must be a *subliminal self.* 'Hidden in the deep of our being is a rubbish-heap as well as a treasure house.' From this subliminal source the works of genius no less than those of deranged personalities well up into consciousness, flashing for a moment in brilliant creativity and 'smouldering again in a lurid and scattered glow'.[1]

It was Myers's 'discovery' of the subliminal self that caused William James to say:

> I cannot but think that the most important step forward that has occurred in psychology since I have been a student of that science is the discovery first made in 1886 that, in certain subjects at least, there is not only the consciousness of the ordinary field, with its usual centre and margin, but an addition thereto in the shape of a set of memories, thoughts and feelings which are extra-marginal and outside of the primary consciousness altogether, but yet must be classed as conscious facts of some sort, able to reveal their presence by unmistakable signs. I call this the most important step forward because, unlike the other advances which psychology has made, this discovery has revealed to us an entirely unsuspected peculiarity in the constitution of human nature. No other step forward which psychology has made can proffer any such claim as this.[2]

Pre-Freudian Clinical Studies

In 1792 Philippe Pinel, in charge of the Bicêtre, had the chains removed from the inmates of his asylum since he no longer believed that insanity was caused by diabolical possession but was a form of mental disease which merited different modes of treatment.[3] His work, and that of Esquirol, was for a time fiercely criticized because of their use of mesmerism, but later studies of hypnotism vindicated the essential truth of Pinel's views.[4] From this time onwards the study

[1] F. W. H. Myers: *Human Personality* (1903 edn) chap. 2.

[2] William James: *The Varieties of Religious Experience* (36th edn 1928) p. 233.

[3] See J. C. Flügel: op. cit. p. 69.

[4] A useful account of how mesmerism (hypnosis) came to be related to psychological techniques is given by Clifford Allen: *Modern Discoveries in Medical Psychology* (1938) pp. 1–60.

of psychopathic cases provided not only a new approach to mental derangement but also an ever-increasing amount of knowledge about the psychology of normal personalities. The fact that patients were relieved by hypnosis of strong emotional tensions indicated the existence of an 'energetic sub-stratum' beneath the level of ordinary awareness. Certain psychologists now became deeply interested in the clinical side of abnormal psychology, and soon a number of outstanding discoveries resulted from the work of Charcot, Janet and Binet in France, and from Breuer and Freud in Vienna. Clinical studies of hysterical patients revealed that

> the mind can [by hypnosis] be so dissociated as to exhibit two or more independent foci of activity, in the sense that synchronous manifestations of different intelligent activities, of one of which the personal consciousness is unaware, can be obtained under experimental and pathological conditions.[1]

In addition to the researches of the Nancy and Paris schools, studies in hysteria, multiple personality, motor automatism and suggestion by James, Sidis, and Morton Prince in America produced a number of highly important theories all of which converged upon that dynamic aspect of the human psyche which is now accepted as 'the unconscious'.

The Twentieth Century

The Psychology of Religion as a separate discipline really emerges from nineteenth-century studies in social psychology, of which Spencer's *Principles* (1876) and Tarde's *Laws of Imitation* (1890) were among the most noteworthy. A little later le Bon in *The Crowd* (1895) described man-in-the-mass as an animal moved by instinctual impulses and passions which swamp all rational considerations, thus furnishing an explanation of why the moral and intellectual level of a crowd is so much lower than that of man as a normal individual. Le Bon's crowd psychology is in part the outcome of practical work by Charcot (who later was to have Janet and Freud among his students), Bernheim and other French psychiatrists. The general convergence of social studies and practical researches into unconscious processes produced, at the turn of the century, the first real psychologies of religion.

Two books laid down the general pattern for future studies,

[1] Pierre Janet quoted by C. Spearman: op. cit. Vol I. p. 377.

Starbuck's *Psychology of Religion* (1899) and William James's *The Varieties of Religious Experience* (1902). Starbuck's book was based on a mass of personal testimony, gathered from many sources, dealing chiefly with the phenomena of religious conversion. In this book, Starbuck attempted to explain the intense emotional conflicts in the religious life of adolescents. William James, in his *Principles of Psychology* (1890), had already shown that he was one of the first psychologists to realize the importance of studying 'abnormal' phenomena as a means of understanding 'normal' personalities. This contributed a good deal to the success of his *Varieties* which was followed two years later by Stanley Hall's *Adolescence* (1904) which contains, *inter alia*, a study of how 'the notion of God' and a moral sense develop among the young.[1] Hall's use of the theory of 'recapitulation' – a theory according to which the individual in his early years repeats swiftly the evolutionary development of man as a species – proved to be a valuable means of relating evolution, psychology and anthropology to the study of religion.[2] Two other books appeared in 1910, Irving King on *The Development of Religion* and E. S. Ames on *The Psychology of Religious Experience*, both of which emphasized the social aspects of religion as well as the anthropological stages of religious development. Other contributions (to which we shall refer more fully later) were made by the French sociologists, Emile Durkheim, Lévy-Bruhl, Hubert and Mauss. Lévy-Bruhl argued that primitive mentality was characterized by 'pre-logical' and 'mystical' forms of thought and that the mind of primitive man and his religion ought not to be assessed in terms such as those which apply to the more civilized levels of mankind.

A very different approach to religion appeared in 1913 when Freud published *Totem and Taboo*, in which he attempted to apply new psychological explanations to primitive cultures, and to anthropology in general. Freud maintained that there was a psychological connexion between the religious practices of primitive man and the behaviour of modern neurotic types. This particular exposition of the relation of psychopathology and primitive cultures was followed by a series of works by psychologists of the Freudian school such as Ernest Jones, Theodore Reik and Oscar Rank. Anthropologists of

[1] In 1917, Hall published *Jesus Christ in the Light of Psychology*, one of the first studies of its kind. This should be compared with Dean Matthews: *The Problem of Christ in the Twentieth Century* (Maurice Lectures: 1949) in order to see how great has been the influence of psychology on modern theology.

[2] See Appendix IV.

the eminence of C. G. Seligman[1] and Bronislaw Malinowski[2] attempted to relate Freudian explanations to matriarchal rather than to patriarchal societies. R. Money-Kyrle[3] offered an alternative psycho-analytical explanation of primitive societies by saying that hate was not, as Freud had contended, primordial and irreducible, but the result of society's frustration of man's natural desires.

The application of psycho-analysis to religion was continued by Freud in such works as *The Future of an Illusion* (1927) and *Moses and Monotheism* (1939). In the meanwhile C. G. Jung, who had for a time collaborated with Freud, presented such a different interpretation of psychology, that his *Psychology of the Unconscious* (1912) marked not only the end of his association with Freud but the beginning of a completely new approach to religion. The Terry Lectures, *Psychology and Religion*, delivered in Yale University in 1938, which are among the most original contributions made in this century, have been followed by a significant number of Jungian studies.

A few writers have tried to relate Adler's *Individual Psychology* (Eng. trans. 1924) to religion because of his emphasis upon the significance of the individual's own constitution. Adler himself in an exchange of views with a Protestant pastor, Ernst Jahn, published in *Religion und Individualpsychologie* (1935), admitted that there was a common ground between religion and Individual Psychology but protested that he was not willing to make his psychology into a Christian exposition since 'the scientific nature of my work must be guarded against the hard and fast criteria of other movements which lie outside science. It cannot possibly make these criteria its own.' [4] Rudolf Allers, however, has been among those who have successfully brought Adler's psychology to bear on individual religious problems, as in his *The Psychology of Character* (1939). G. W. Allport in *The Individual and his Religion* (1951) stressed the fact that religion is the most satisfactory means of unifying the separate activities of man as an individual, and at the same time strongly emphasized the need to relate personality to environment and belief. None the less, despite many outstanding contributions, contemporary studies tend either to be somewhat highly specialized studies of

[1] See *Anthropology and Psychology* (1924).
[2] See *Sex and Repression in Primitive Society* (1926).
[3] See *Aspasia – or the Future of A-morality* (1932).
[4] Quoted by Lewis Way: *Alfred Adler – An Introduction to his Psychology* (1956) p. 51.

individual aspects of religion or else elaborations of William James, Freud and Jung.

Psychology and Comparative Religion

Interest in world religions was stimulated in the nineteenth century by comparative studies of Indo-Germanic languages. Up to that time the religious ideas of the West had been confined to the religions of classical antiquity and Christianity. In the seventeenth century, Lord Herbert of Cherbury advanced the view that the common 'notions' of religion are apprehended 'by human instinct'. John Locke maintained that the human understanding was not capable of apprehending the true nature of reality and that it needed to be supplemented by faith. Speaking generally, the English Deists, who supported natural religion as against revealed religion (a distinction introduced by St Thomas Aquinas), attempted to find some underlying element common to all known religions, an inquiry which was stimulated by the information which missionary enterprises brought back from newly opened territories overseas.

In 1723, Father Joseph Lafitau S.J., as the result of a study of the similarities which he had observed between the rites of American aborigines, classical Europe and the Catholic Church, suggested that the 'original' religion was a universal form of nature worship. Another suggestion in the same century came from Charles-François Dupuis who said that behind such figures as Bacchus, Osiris, Mithras and Christ, there was a common theme derived from sun worship. But it was not until Benjamin Constant in France and Christoph Meiners in Germany became interested in this subject that we find any really concerted attempt to deal with the psychological features of world religions. Constant and Meiners both agreed that the absolute distinction between 'heathen' religions and Christianity could not be fully maintained, that psychologically the various religions seemed to have more in common than their theological differences suggested. The general result was that German studies in the nineteenth century came to the conclusion that all religions are expressions of a primordial revelation. For instance, Schleiermacher, who represents one of the most important contributors to the psychology of religion in its formative stages, held that religion was not a dogmatic system directed mainly to the intellect of believers, nor yet a corpus of precepts addressed to the will; religion arose primarily from a simple, elementary feeling of dependence upon God. By basing religion on feeling and the yearnings of the soul, Schleiermacher furnished a common basis for the religions of mankind which have to be viewed, each in its own way, as a manifestation of man's feeling of dependence on a Power other than himself or society.

The introduction of the comparative method into the study of religion proceeded upon the assumption that practices and ideas which originated in the remote past continue to be operative in the present because they spring from impulses common to mankind and relate to concepts which are as valid in the modern world as they were in elementary forms of society. Knowledge about the psychology of world religions was extended still further by the successful attempts of Herbert Spencer to apply the newly formulated theory of evolution to psychology in general. Furthermore, Alfred Wallace and Charles Darwin by stressing the vital part played by evolution in mental processes enabled psychologists to view the behavioural processes of children, primitive peoples and animals as part of a general development, though the attempt to relate the psychology of man to the behaviour of lower creatures provoked Jean Henri Fabre to remark that 'man is not a higher sort of insect'.

Later developments are very much indebted to the works of E. B. Tylor[1] and William Robertson Smith,[2] both of whom inspired James Frazer to produce a stream of great works of which *The Golden Bough* (originally published in two volumes in 1890) and *Folklore in the Old Testament* (three volumes in 1918) are the best known. In *The Gorgon's Head* (1927) Frazer says of Robertson Smith's use of the comparative method:

> The idea of regarding the religions of the world not dogmatically but historically – in other words, not as systems of truth or falsehood to be demonstrated or refuted, but as phenomena of consciousness to be studied like any other aspect of human nature – is one which seems hardly to have suggested itself before the nineteenth century. Now when, laying aside as irrelevant to the purpose in hand the question of the truth or falsehood of religious beliefs, and the question of the wisdom or folly of religious practices, we examine side by side the religions of the different races and ages, we find that, while they differ from each other in many particulars, the resemblances between them are numerous and fundamental, and that they mutually illustrate and explain each other, the distinctly stated faith and circumstantial ritual of one race often clearing up ambiguities in the faith and practice of other races. Thus the comparative study of religion soon forces on us the conclusion that the

[1] *Primitive Culture* (1871). [2] *Religion of the Semites* (1889).

> course of religious evolution has been, up to a certain point, very similar among all men, and that no one religion, at all events in its earlier stages, can be fully understood without a comparison of it with many others.[1]

Both Robertson Smith and Frazer found that they were able to reach an understanding of rituals, institutions and practices in Semitic religion by the use of analogies drawn from non-Semitic sources. Our present interest, however, is not in the actual anthropological details but in the impulses which underlie them. As Frazer himself said in explaining his reasons for writing *The Golden Bough*:

> Recent researches into the early history of man have revealed the essential similarity with which, under many superficial differences, the human mind has elaborated its first crude philosophy of life. If we can show that a barbarous custom like that of the priesthood of Nemi, has existed elsewhere; if we can prove that these motives have operated widely, perhaps universally, in human society, producing in varied circumstances a variety of institutions specifically different but generically alike . . . then we may fairly infer that at a remote age the same motives gave birth to the priesthood of Nemi.[2]

What explanation, we may ask, can be offered for such universal (or near universal) practices? The most immediate explanation would seem to be that of cultural diffusion, but as we pointed out earlier on, cultural diffusions do not deny the existence of universal psychological factors in the human make-up. Many of the basic similarities in religion and culture are due to the common psychological nature of man. 'Mankind moves forward but Man remains ever the same.'[3] Man has had and continues to have needs, not all of them physical, which are common to all men everywhere. It is because of this that psychology is able to offer explanations of world-wide religious practices both as the expression of, and at the same time the means of satisfying these vital common needs.

[1] J. G. Frazer: *The Gorgon's Head* (1927) pp. 281–2.
[2] Frazer: op. cit.: abridged edition (1925) p. 2.
[3] Goethe quoted by Professor Herbert Kühn: *On the Tracks of Prehistoric Man* (1958) p. 16.

Chapter III

THE ORIGINS OF RELIGION

The psychologist approaches this matter somewhat differently from the theologian, the historian or the anthropologist, although he cannot proceed very far without borrowing substantially from all of them. The psychologist is not concerned solely with religious events, customs and artefacts, but with religion as the expression of human needs and experiences.

> Experience shows that religions are in no sense conscious constructions but that they arise from the natural life of the unconscious psyche and somehow give adequate expression to it. This explains their universal distribution and their enormous influence on humanity throughout history which would be incomprehensible if religious symbols were not at the very least truths of man's psychological nature. . . . Religions are psychotherapeutic systems in the truest sense of the word . . . they express the whole range of the psychic problem in powerful images.[1]

In other words, the psychologist when considering the origins of religion is concerned with what takes place in the human soul in so far as he can deduce such evidence from anthropology, studies of child psychology, dreams, complexes, the neuroses of adult minds and general experiences. The limits of the psychologist's endeavours were indicated some years ago by James H. Leuba:

> As to the psychologist, he may regard his task as completed when he has pointed out the several possible origins of the god-ideas, the characteristics of each, and the nature of the general causes which determine the dominance of particular gods. . . . It is for the anthropologist and the historian to discover what in any particular case has actually happened . . . and to determine the origin or origins of any particular god.[2]

It is plain from these two quotations that no one discipline can offer a complete and all-embracive explanation. We ourselves are under no

[1] Jung: 'The Soul and Death': *The Structure and Dynamics of the Psyche*: Collected Works: Vol. 8 (1961) par. 805.

[2] J. H. Leuba: *A Psychological Study of Religion; its Origin, Function and Future* (1912) pp. 99 ff.

compulsion to invent a psychological theory of origins, it will be sufficient if we indicate some of the ways in which man has responded from prehistoric to historic times to the 'mystery' of existence.

Religion and the Primitive Mind

Modern anthropology has been able to show how comparatively recent is the emergence of the modern mind. Professor Gordon Childe[1] said that the modern mind came into existence within the last six or seven thousand years as the result of a change-over from a food-gathering to a food-producing economy, when 'a new type of urban civilization based upon industry and commerce' appeared within the Fertile Crescent. Previous to that time mankind lived for untold centuries in small nomadic tribes whose main activity was that of food-gathering.[2]

A particularly important comparison between the primitive and the civilized mind was presented by the French sociologists, Durkheim and Lévy-Bruhl. This French school rejected the assumption that the mind of man, like his body, is the result of a continuous development over millions of years. Lévy-Bruhl contended that the mind of primitive man differs so markedly from that of civilized man that the laws of logic and the principles of psychology are quite inapplicable, the mind of primitive man being 'pre-logical' and 'mystical'. By pre-logical, Lévy-Bruhl meant that primitive man had no aversion to accepting logical contradictions. The term 'mystique' is used to indicate that primitive man was conscious of being subject to occult powers which varied in their operation from object to object and circumstance to circumstance, powers that were not perceptible by the senses but were none the less immediate and real in human experience. These two concepts are closely related to yet another important concept – *représentations collectives.* These *représentations* are common to all members of a social group, being transmitted from generation to generation, and, by imposing themselves upon the individuals within a community, arouse in them sentiments of rever-

[1] *New Light on the Most Ancient East* (1934).

[2] Recent excavations at Jericho and elsewhere show that pioneer farmers were active in south-west Asia as early as 7000 B.C. See K. M. Kenyon: *Digging up Jericho* (1957). A fusion of this food-growing activity with the food-gathering forms of culture coincides with the emergence of the Earth Goddess as a distinct expression of the powers associated with fertility. There is an abundance of Palaeolithic and Neolithic evidence for the worship of the Mother Goddess – Neolithic figurines having been found in early farming cultures of the fifth and sixth millennia B.C. See Paolo Graziosi: *Palaeolithic Art* (1960).

ence and adoration. But we must observe that *représentations* for Lévy-Bruhl do not mean what they mean in modern psychology where the term is primarily an intellectual concept; Lévy-Bruhl uses the term to designate those occasions which, in the experience of a primitive community, give rise to such intensities of emotional excitement that their subsequent representation in dance and ritual forms 'recapitulates' the original circumstances and evokes the same kind of emotional response. Such situations are included among those events which are described as 'mystical'. It is the operation of these pre-logical and mystical elements in the life of primitive man that differentiates primitive from modern mentality.[1]

Since these views present a strong challenge to arguments previously advanced, we have to ask what objections can be offered in reply? Perhaps the most important objection is that these French sociologists made the mistake of basing their conclusions on cultures which have subsequently been shown to be advanced stages of society or else degenerate forms of one-time higher levels of civilized life. The views of British anthropologists present a markedly different picture. Murphy and Rivers, for instance, have stated in quite other terms the difference between what may be called 'the generalized mind' and 'the collective mentality', the former term being that employed by the British, and the latter by the French schools. Professor Murphy described the 'generalized mind' in the following passage:

> the mind of man at all points of its history is generically the same. The primitive mind and the civilized mind are earlier and later stages of the same developing thing. They are generically connected: and cultured thought is a specific descendant, more highly differentiated and more deeply integrated, of a generalized and primitive type of thought. The mind of man is the subject of evolution, as well as his body: and, as the brain, the organ of the mind, can be traced through well defined steps of development from that of the animal up to the brain of civilized man, so the evolution of mind, could it be traced, would be found to be substantially continuous from the animal and ape-like mind of the generalized sub-human type, through truly human primitive forms, onward to the most refined modern mentality. . . . However different they may seem from each other, as the raw green blade from the golden head of corn, these earlier mental phenomena are regarded as elementary forms of the

[1] Lévy-Bruhl later abandoned his distinction between logical and pre-logical aspects of primitive thinking because of the amount of logical thought to be found among modern 'primitives'. See the posthumous publication: *Les Carnets de Lucien Lévy-Bruhl* (1949).

later, into which they have developed by a process of continuous evolution.[1]

W. H. R. Rivers stated the case as follows:

> According to the French school, the work of practically the whole body of English anthropologists suffers from the radical defect that it supposes social institutions to have arisen in consequence of the realization of primitive ideas logically akin to our own: that our social ideas have been moulded by long ages of the evolution which has produced our present condition of society, and Durkheim and his disciples reject the view that they have been operative at all stages of man's history.[2]

But the most formidable criticisms of the French school were advanced by Fr Wilhelm Schmidt of Vienna, some of whose criticisms are contained in the following lengthy quotation:

> In the first place, Lévy-Bruhl nowhere gives a scientifically accurate definition . . . of what he means by 'primitive'. Secondly, we look in vain in his works for the slightest indication of any arrangement of the various groups of peoples which he mentions in their historical sequence: in this respect he indulges in a wild confusion, to be equalled only in the writings of the oldest Evolutionists. Thirdly, and in consequence of this, he fails to make the least attempt at a historical arrangement of the several stages of pre-logical thought, or any investigation of the question whether there is more pre-logicality in the earlier or later stages, or whether it is more marked in the one or the other. . . . Fourthly, he completely neglects the fact that there are plenty of pre-logical states to be found even in the civilizations of Europe and America (witness our fashions, our 'movements', our superstitions, our prejudices, yes, and the theories and ideas of certain expositors of 'exact' sciences); . . . And, fifthly, it is astonishing how much sheer ignorance he is capable of displaying in such pronouncements as the following: that primitive man comprehends *nothing* as we do: that he refers everything to a *mystical* (i.e. a non-natural) origin: that he *never* regards sickness or death as due to natural causes: that he does *nothing* without magical means: that he derives *everything* from a magical force: and that he knows *no* difference between man and beasts.[3]

Parts of this quotation appear to be almost as sweeping as the statements which it criticizes, but Jung in his chapter on 'Archaic Man'[4] agrees that primitive man was no more illogical than modern man. There seems, says Jung, to be nothing to indicate that primitive man

[1] John Murphy: *Primitive Man – His Essential Quest* (1927) p. 88.
[2] W. H. R. Rivers: *Psychology and Ethnology* (1926) p. 36.
[3] Wilhelm Schmidt: *The Origin and Growth of Religion:* Eng. trans. H. J. Rose (1931) pp. 133–4.
[4] See *Modern Man in Search of a Soul* (1936) pp. 143–74.

is any less logical than modern man, his psychic functions are essentially the same as those of modern man, the chief differences are in the primary assumptions and in the areas of consciousness over which he is able to maintain a concentrated attention. Primitive man dispenses with intellectual processes at every possible opportunity because thinking is intolerably tiring to the primitive mind. (It seems also to be a burden to a large proportion of modern society whose 'intellectual processes' show a persistent desire to avoid any prolonged mental effort.) The best way of avoiding intellectual fatigue is to become motor-active – hence the importance and widespreadness of ritual gestures and magical acts – ritualistic activity always precedes theological exposition. This argument is supported by an important distinction advanced by Varendonch.[1]

Varendonch distinguished between Reduplicative and Synthetical Memory. The first refers to that kind of memory in which a long sequence of individual experiences forms a chronological series which the primitive mind can repeat 'by heart' without difficulty, particularly when the sequence is couched in rhythmical form. Reduplicative memory is still operative in modern man, being the last form of memory to disappear under the influence of drugs, age or mental derangement, a fact indicative of its early appearance in human development. On the other hand, synthetical memory proceeds by classification of individual experiences and thus represents a much later stage of intellectual development. Primitive religions show the operation of reduplicative memory in rites whose repeated physical gestures and repetitive words are the results of man's desire to avoid the fatigue experienced in synthetical memory. This fact is clearly supported in the life of small children who find it easier to learn items expressed in repetitive verbal forms than subjects calling for logical integration of newly acquired knowledge. The multiplication table is easier to learn than to apply.

We may sum up this section briefly by saying that if the evolutionary development of the human brain has its corresponding development in human mentality, then this process may be taken to indicate a basic mental development which has shown itself over hundreds of thousands of years in a wide variety of activities of which religious practices and concepts are an essential part. Some of these we shall now proceed to discuss.

[1] J. Varendonch: *Evolution of the Conscious Faculties* (1923).

Tribal Religion

The connexion between religion and the life of the tribe has been discussed from many angles. Gilbert Murray[1] says that there are levels of tribal life at which there is no personal god, but that later on men came to believe that the blood of a totemic animal is identical with the 'life' of the tribe and this led to some personalized form of the tribal *mana*. The idea of personal gods grows in definiteness as man's own personality becomes more and more unified and his tribal life more closely organized. When several tribes are incorporated in a larger grouping, the local or tribal gods are united in a larger concept of deity. Durkheim pursued a somewhat similar idea when he said that tribal solidarity leads to a deification of the tribal 'life'.

Social groupings show at least three distinctive stages in the history of culture and religion. The first stage is that of the 'food-gatherers', the second, that of the 'food-growers', and the third, a combination of food-gatherers and food-growers. E. Washburn Hopkins[2] contended that there is an intimate connexion between the kind of early society and the kind of religion it practises. He suggested that among African people at the level of hunting or food-gathering, religion is of an impulsive, changeful and unreflective character and corresponds to the stage of fetichism. Later, at the more settled food-raising level, religion shows a greater stability due to more ample opportunities for reflection. At the tribal level a hierarchical development takes place: 'The bigger the state, the bigger the god compounded of various gods: the bigger the god's province, the less confined his activities. His comprehensiveness tends to make him more abstract.'[3] This theory is generally but not universally applicable; for instance, it has been shown that although the gods of Australian aborigines exhibit some degree of definiteness and even some indication of a presiding spirit, yet their social patterns do not in any way correspond to the distinctions between food-gatherers, food-raisers and societies which represent a combination of both.

Mana

The concept of *mana* is so important for the origins of religion that we must see how the term came into use and also in what way such a con-

[1] Gilbert Murray: *The Rise of the Greek Epic* (1924) p. 62.
[2] E. W. Hopkins: *The History of Religions* (1918).
[3] op. cit. p. 25.

cept was believed to operate. Professor Mircea Eliade, discussing 'The Structure and Morphology of the Sacred', says:

> The unknown and the extraordinary are disturbing epiphanies; they indicate the presence of something *other* than the natural; the presence, or at least the call of that something. A particularly cunning animal, anything novel, any monstrosity – all these are as clearly marked out as a man who is exceptionally ugly, neurotic or shut off from the rest of the community by any sort of distinguishing mark . . . (whether natural or acquired). Such examples may help us to understand the Melanesian idea of *mana* from which some authors have thought it possible to trace the origins of every religious phenomenon. *Mana* is for the Melanesians, that mysterious but active power which belongs to certain people and generally to the souls of the dead and all spirits.[1]

The concept was first introduced to Western thought in 1891 by Bishop R. H. Codrington who, in his book on the Melanesians, stated that he believed that the concept *mana* was common to the whole Pacific. He defined the term as:

> a force altogether distinct from physical power which acts in all kinds of ways for good and evil, and which it is of the greatest advantage to possess or control. . . . It is a power or influence, not physical, and in a way supernatural; but it shows itself in physical force, or in any kind of power or excellence which a man possesses. This *mana* is not fixed in anything and can be conveyed in almost anything; but spirits, whether disembodied or supernatural beings, have it and can impart it; and it essentially belongs to personal beings to originate it, though it may act through the medium of water, or a stone or a bone.[2]

If a man is successful as a fighter or a hunter, or if his animals multiply or the plants he is cultivating flourish, it is because he has *mana* in himself, or his weapons or tools have *mana* or the garden has *mana*. If a man sees a stone which seems to him to have an unusual shape, and if he buries it in his field and a good crop follows, then it is because the stone has *mana*. Similarly if a man is able to emulate his predecessor who was judged to be a great man, it is because he has the same *mana*. *Mana* is something that is to be found both in human beings and in things, and it can be transmitted by man to things, or by things to things.

The religion of the Melanesians seems to have been largely devoted to obtaining this power of *mana*, but *mana* is now known to be operative in a much more extended realm than Melanesian religion, it

[1] Mircea Eliade: *Patterns in Comparative Religion* (1958) p. 19.
[2] R. H. Codrington: *The Melanesians: Studies in their Anthropology and Folklore* (1891) pp. 118–19.

plays a considerable part, under different names, in the religions of many other areas. For instance, among the Iroquois it is called *orenda*, with the Sioux it is *wakai*, and with the Algonquin it is *manitu*. In Queensland the Kabi tribesmen have a similar concept which they call *manngur*. Generally speaking these terms refer to a mysterious, wonder-working element that can produce results both creative and destructive. Since the term, or its equivalents, plays such a prominent part in early forms of religion there has been a considerable debate as to whether religion has its origin in some such concept, whether *mana* precedes animism and what is its connexion with magic. Pringle-Pattison, discussing the history of religion, said that

> The history of religion may legitimately be treated as a continuous development from the vague *mana* beliefs of primitive savagery. Progress will consist in the attainment of clearer and worthier conceptions of the nature of the power(s) with which we have to do.[1]

A somewhat similar point of view was advanced by MM. Hubert and Mauss who, in their *Mélanges d'Histoire des Religions* (1909), identified the 'sacred' with *mana* as the most elementary of all religious forms known to us. It is obvious that such a concept is fundamental to very early forms of religion, but we have not yet asked how man came to believe in such a power, or to form such a concept?

Primitive man seems to have conceived of everything within his environment as being a centre of certain forces. If he picked up something that was heavy, or attempted to push something that was difficult to move, or touched something that gave a strong impression of being solid, or saw the swift movements of rushing water, avalanches and falling trees, all such physical experiences caused him to compare these forces with the movements and tensions in his own body. Indeed, it may be doubted whether at an early stage he was able to make a clear distinction between forces outside and forces within his own body. Carveth Read says that there is an *Einfühlung* or empathy between man and the movements and sounds emitted by things. Man responds to the moaning of the wind and the whispering of the sea, their 'voices' endow them with a life which R. R. Marett (see section on 'Animism and Animatism') has called 'animatism', a belief that every object is actuated by a life that is of the same kind as our own. From such 'sympathetic' thinking, Carveth Read suggests that it is but a step to the concept of *mana*.[2]

[1] A. Seth Pringle-Pattison: *Studies in the Philosophy of Religion* (1930) p. 29.
[2] Carveth Read: *Man and his Superstitions* (1920).

Jung, when discussing Robert Mayer's theory of the conservation of *energy*,[1] asks how did this new idea thrust itself into consciousness with such elemental force? To which Jung replies that the idea of energy was a 'primordial image' that emerged from the collective unconscious.[2] Jung argues that some such concept as 'primitive energetics' underlies religion in all parts of the world; it is that 'universal magical power' which is behind all the dynamistic religions which Tylor and Frazer mistakenly interpreted as animism. The power-concept of *mana* was not, says Jung, thought of in terms of souls or spirits. In a chapter on 'Mana-Personality' Jung says:

> Primitive man does not analyse and does not work out why another is superior to him. If another is cleverer or stronger than he, then he has *mana*, he is possessed of a stronger power. . . . Historically this *mana*-personality evolves into the hero and the godlike being whose earthly form is the priest.[3]

Kings as late as the eighteenth century were supposed to have some such power of 'touch' by which to cure disease. 'Historically the *mana*-personality is always in possession of the secret name or some special esoteric knowledge.' Jung goes on to say that men in later times instead of identifying the self with the *mana*-personality, as primitive men tried to do, concretized it as an extra-mundane 'Father-in-Heaven'.

Discussing the 'primitive conception of libido' [4] Jung argues that *mana* is not something that 'refers to things that call forth reverent wonder, respect or love – but rather to what is effective, powerful and creative'. The primitive conception of *mana*, says Jung, seems, therefore, to be an initial stage of our general conception of psychic energy; this energy at the personification stage is seen as animism and so is an important prior condition of the God-idea, and perhaps the most primitive of all such concepts.

Magic

Magic belongs to very early stages of human development but it is difficult to establish its place in the evolution of religion. Tylor, and

[1] Robert Mayer: *Kleinere Schriften und Briefe* (1893) p. 213.

[2] See A. O. Lovejoy: 'The Fundamental Concept of the Primitive Philosophy': *The Monist* XVI (1906) pp. 361 ff., where the idea of 'primitive energetics' is discussed.

[3] Jung: *Two Essays on Analytical Psychology*: Collected Works. Vol. 7 (1953) p. 231 f.

[4] Jung: *Contributions to Analytical Psychology* (1928) pp. 70 ff.

Spencer and Gillen, all relegated magic to the background, believing animism to be of far greater importance. Frazer believed that there was an absolute difference between magic and religion, saying that Australian aborigines possessed magic but hardly a religion. This opinion has proved, on two grounds, to be ill-founded: (1) recent studies have shown that many Australian aborigines did in actual fact worship sky-gods, and (2) modern anthropology shows that between belief in *mana* and belief in spirits there is a succession of intermediate stages among which magic would naturally find a place.

One of the earliest and most valuable expositions of magic was written by J. H. King,[1] whose theory depends upon a distinction which he made between two kinds of 'power' – the *impersonal* (what is generally meant by physical energy) and the *mental* (as seen in man and animals). From the first of these two kinds of power man arrived at the practice of magic, and from the second at a belief in spirits – the magical being the earlier form of belief in physical energies. Human experience at all stages is subject to unpredictable interruptions by *impersonal* powers which men describe as good or bad luck. Magic arises from situations involving 'luck' and is, according to King, the first germ of religion. But how did magical practices as such come into being? R. R. Marett suggested that primitive man when confronted with startling or extraordinary situations expressed his emotional reactions by vivid physical gestures. These gestures tended to be repeated whenever these situations recurred, and so became, by a process of repetition and association, a sort of formal technique by which man sought to avert some danger or to satisfy some urgent need.

Marett's explanation agrees with King's in stressing the importance of man's psycho-physical reactions to the unusual and the unexpected, but King's explanation omitted all reference to the collective aspect of magical activities. This omission was repaired by MM. Hubert and Mauss[2] who argued that magic like religion is the expression of a collective consciousness; mass emotions tend to endow physical acts with powers believed to be capable of satisfying collective needs.

If simplicity is a characteristic of primitive thought then it seems probable that magic precedes animism in the development of reli-

[1] J. H. King: *The Supernatural: Origin, Nature and Evolution* (1892) 2 vols.
[2] See *Exquisse d'une théorie générale de la Magie: Année Sociologique* Vol. VII (1902–1903) pp. 1–140.

gion. Wundt, however, while he accepted this statement, argued that the concept of the soul is older than that of magic because it arises directly out of two of the most striking of all human experiences, namely the phenomena of death and dreams.[1] The order of development would seem to be, the concept of the soul, the concept of *mana*, the practice of magic and the rise of animatism followed by animism. This sequence is, however, open to objection by those who maintain that animism precedes magic, but whatever the order, it is clear that magical practices played a prominent part in the earliest stages of religion and continue to do so even among civilized peoples, many of whom still believe that there is another 'causal' order than that which is commonly described as scientific.

Animatism and Animism

E. B. Tylor in *Primitive Culture* (1871) expounded the idea that Animism was the most primitive form of religion, a theory which James Frazer also adopted. Tylor said that man very early came to believe that all things, including so-called inert objects, were animated by personal 'souls' which assumed human shapes in dreams and visions. Even at primitive levels man realized that two things belonged to him as well as his body – life and a 'double'. But Tylor did not think it necessary to make a distinction between an all-pervading spirit and individual souls which animate individual things.

Tylor argued that once man had learned to distinguish between his body and some phantom being or 'double' it was but a step to allying this 'double' with the concept of life, thus producing the concept of a personal soul. Marett contended that the notion of individual spirits is really too clearly defined a concept to be a satisfactory 'minimum definition of religion': 'Savage religion is something not so much thought out as danced out, that, in other words, it develops under conditions, psychological and sociological, which favour emotional or motor processes, whereas ideation remains relatively in abeyance.' [2] Something less intellectualized was needed than Tylor's animism, and so it was found necessary to postulate a pre-animistic stage in religion. Such a stage would correspond either to the *mana*-stage or to what Marett called Animatism. Under this term Marett introduced a distinction between treating objects as if they were infused with life (animatism) and the animistic belief that

[1] Wundt: *Mythus und Religion* (1905–1909) pp. 78 ff.
[2] R. R. Marett: *The Threshold of Religion* (1914) p. 31.

natural objects had each an individual soul. But whatever theories may be advanced for the actual development from the *mana*-stage to animism, we need to notice that 'in the remote times (which can still be observed among primitives living to-day) the main body of psychic life was apparently in human and in non-human objects; it was projected as we should say now'.[1] It is this fact, says Jung, that may be taken as the psychological explanation of the theory of animism.

Totemism

Totemism both as a concept and as a practice is exemplified in the tribal customs of North American and Australian peoples who form societies made up of groups united by kinship (real or imaginary), each clan being distinguished from other clans by the name and worship of some species of animal or plant. This object (whether animal or vegetable) is thought of as being related to the clan in a particular way, and so is the subject of a religious emotion as well as of a protecting taboo. As examples of totemic objects we may cite the Crane, Bear, Marten and the Wolf which are among the most representative totems of North American Ojibwas and Iroquois. Totemism is a widely distributed practice. In Australia, in West Africa and in India (among peoples who are probably of Dravidian origin) totemism is a long-established form of religion, as it is also in the islands of Polynesia.

The actual origin of this practice has been variously explained. Spencer and Gillen suggested that it arose as an explanation of conception and childbirth, the totemic power being thought of as that which fertilizes the female body. Andrew Lang associated the origin of totemism with the *mana*-like qualities of the tribal name, while Durkheim considered totemism to be the expression of an impersonal force thought of as resident in some totemic cult object. Professor Murphy advanced a similar explanation of totemism as an extension of the *mana* principle.

> As a primitive religious system . . . it springs from the food interest, for the totem is the food animal or plant regarded as mysterious but as beneficent. The conception of being of one blood with the totem, or of one flesh, rises up into the sense of kinship to it . . . the totem-divinity is the father or ancestor of the clan.[2]

---

[1] Jung: *Psychology and Religion: West and East*: Collected Works: Vol. 11 (1958) p. 83. [2] John Murphy: *Lamps of Anthropology* (1943) p. 4.

Our interest in totemism at this stage arises from W. Robertson Smith's belief that totemism was the starting point of all religions.[1] It was, he suggested, the root of all Semitic religions and of the faith which is embraced by the most civilized nations of the world. Robertson Smith said that it was believed among Semitic peoples that the blood of the victim offered in sacrifices was the same blood as that of the god to whom the sacrifice was made. The flesh of such a victim might not be eaten except at a communal meal upon ritual occasions. This suggestion was followed up by F. B. Jevons[2] who said that if each tribe has its own totemic deity, then each tribe was a believer in a sort of tribal monotheism, a suggestion which will be discussed from another point of view in the section on 'Original Monotheism'.

Nature Worship

James Frazer maintained that a very large part of religion in its earliest stages was based upon a personification of Nature.[3] This worship had a mythology which, according to Max Müller, came into being because of a confusion of primitive language.[4] Primitive man had individual names for individual objects but in many cases no general class names for objects of the same species, so that names tended to get confused and this with the personification of *mana* objects eventually led to a combination of several gods in one and the separation of the one into the many. Such a process is related by Müller to his three-fold classification of cult objects: (1) things that can be grasped by the hands (fetiches); (2) things that can be partially grasped but are too large to be lifted, such as large natural objects (nature gods); (3) things that cannot be grasped at all, sky, sun, stars which become the Greater Gods above whom there stands the Infinite. This conception of an all-presiding power arose from man's consciousness of powers within himself which exceed those of

[1] In spite of the extensive areas over which totemistic practices have been known to operate it cannot be claimed that religion necessarily originated in totemism because there are large areas of the world which seem not to have had any form of totemism but which, none the less, have religions of one kind or another.

[2] F. B. Jevons: *The Idea of God in Early Religions* (1910).

[3] J. G. Frazer: *The Worship of Nature* (1926).

[4] 'For him [Müller], myth is neither a transformation of history into fabulous legend, nor is it fable accepted as history: and just as certainly it does not spring directly from the contemplation of the great forms and powers of nature. What we call myth is, for him, something conditioned and negotiated by the agency of language; it is in fact, the product of a basic shortcoming, an inherent weakness of language.' Ernst Cassirer: *Language and Myth* (1960) pp. 3–4.

ordinary waking consciousness, and on this basis, Müller argued that man produced 'a psychological religion'. Perhaps the best comment upon the place of Nature Worship in the development of religion is that which Frazer himself offers in his own Introduction to *The Worship of Nature*:

> The mind of man refuses to acquiesce in the phenomena of sense. By an instinctive, an irresistible impulse it is driven to seek for something beyond, something which it assumes to be more real and abiding, than the shifting phantasmagoria of this sensible world. This search and this assumption are not peculiar to philosophers; they are shared in varying degrees by every man and woman born into the world.

* * *

Two other developments, Ancestor Worship and Astral Religion, are sometimes advanced as explanations of the origin of religion. Both are important, but the first plays only a limited part in the religions of some primitive peoples, while the latter represents a somewhat late stage of religious beliefs.

* * *

An Original Monotheism

The idea that primitive man believed in an original form of monotheism was first adumbrated by Max Müller and later developed by Father Wilhelm Schmidt. It has been argued that early man had an idea of the Infinite because 'everything of which his senses cannot perceive a limit is to a primitive savage or to any man in an early stage of intellectual activity, *unlimited* or *infinite*'.[1] This idea bears a close resemblance to that crude sense of mystery which primitive man feels in the presence of what Otto called the *numinous*.[2] But these cruder feelings of the weird and the uncanny were not likely to include for primitive man those other aspects of the *numinous* which Otto describes as majestic, sublime, the 'wholly other' (*das ganz Andere*) or 'The Holy'. The appreciation of these attributes belongs to much more highly developed levels of religious consciousness. But this in no way lessens the fundamental part which the *numinous* plays in primitive religions, for a sense of the mysterious and the awe-ful is among the earliest known forms of human experience.

Schmidt's argument for an original monotheism rests in part upon

[1] See Andrew Lang: *Custom and Myth* (1904) p. 30.
[2] See Rudolf Otto: *The Idea of the Holy* (1928).

man's sense of the mysterious and the infinite, and in part upon his refusal to apply the theory of evolution to religion. From long studies of primitive peoples Schmidt showed that religious developments are not always nor necessarily linked with stages of social evolution but that among some of the earliest known forms of society there were to be found 'high' forms of religious belief. To borrow a phrase from Andrew Lang – there was among Low Races a belief in High Gods. Schmidt's argument (reduced to a few words) is that what he calls 'das höchtes Wesen' was not some concept that was the result of evolutionary development from earlier forms of religion but the recognition by 'the ethnologically oldest people' of some form of exalted deity. By identifying 'the ethnologically oldest peoples' with Pygmies and similar peoples, Schmidt seriously impaired his argument. Modern anthropologists have pointed out that the Pygmies, the lowest of the Amerindians, the Eskimos and the Ainus, are ethnologically no older than the 'tall peoples' of the same stock. But if we disregard the ethnological aspect there seems to be some weight in the argument that a form of monotheism began to emerge early on in the history of mankind. There is reason to suppose that primitive man's belief in High Gods, or in some form of localized monotheism, has its modern parallel in the religious development of young children who associate a Big Being with Big Things.

We have now to refer to the place of fear and fascination in religion.

The Numinous

Man, long before he was able to make any intellectual explanation of his experiences, was aware that there were situations which aroused feelings of fear, awe, reverence, repulsion and attraction, intuitions of the Mysterious and the Inexplicable; the sort of thing which, at many removes, we find in Jacob's experience of sleeping at Bethel, 'How dreadful is this place!' Tens of thousands of years before Jacob fell asleep with a stone for his pillow, men had known what it was to have a feeling of the Awe-ful. As Dr G. F. Moore puts it:

> in a thousand ways the primitive is made aware that besides his fellow-men, friends or enemies, besides the animals he pursues or which pursue him, in short, besides the things he is familiar with or more or less understands, there are around him other things that are outside his understanding as they are beyond his foresight or control.[1]

[1] G. F. Moore: *The Birth and Growth of Religion* (1923) p. 9, quoted E. O. James: *The Beginnings of Religion*: Grey Arrow edn (1958) p. 30.

In other words, there is a vivid recognition of the difference between the familiar and the mysterious, between the Natural and Supernatural.

This feeling of the difference between the familiar and the mysterious is the basis of the most important religious concept of modern times – the Numinous. Otto's numinous, this feeling of *Something-Other-Than*, is a fact of experience. And it exercises a tremendous influence over the primitive mind – but not over the primitive mind only. The sense of the mysterious has not evaporated even in the most highly technical forms of urbanized society. What this numinous Something is we cannot fully define or describe. It is not only *tremendum*, it is also described as *fascinans*. Like fear itself, it is accompanied by the opposite feeling of love and attraction. Repulsion and fascination are the twin poles of man's reactions to the unfamiliar, the tremendous, the majestic and the awesome. Religion, however many other definitions may be forthcoming, is man's 'effective desire to be in right relations with a sacred transcendental order controlling human destinies and natural events – which finds expression in a prescribed system of ritual and belief'.[1] The human soul is so constituted as to be able to respond to the mysterious wherever it may be felt. That the mysterious may appear to take on different forms in different orders of society does not alter the fact that man knows what it is to experience situations of Something-other-than which arouse in him reactions of fear, fascination, wonder and awe.

Résumé

We may now make a brief résumé of what we have said about the psychological factors involved in the origin of religion.

Religion is an active element in human life at all levels of development because it is directly related to basic human needs. These needs are not wholly physical because life is never entirely a practical affair. The fact that primitive man sought for non-physical means of satisfying many of his basic needs implies a belief in the existence of spiritual agencies.

Psychologically man does not always live on the same level of consciousness. In sleep he becomes vividly aware of another life which is apparently independent of his physical activity. It is reasonable to suppose that primitive man, being ignorant of the psycho-

[1] E. O. James: op. cit. p. 30.

logical structure of his own nature, arrived at his belief in the existence of the soul or psyche not from dream experiences only but from some such practical consideration as the distinction between a body that breathes and a body that does not. This primeval distinction was in the course of many centuries endowed with a rich vocabulary, a vocabulary which shows that man from very early times identified breath and blood with soul, psyche and life.

Man's religious consciousness was extended by his awareness of an *empathy* between the interior forces of his own life and the things of the external world; by this means the things of the natural world were endowed with individual forces or souls which man came to think of as personified beings, thus providing himself with the first assembly of gods. Added to this his experience of the large and the immeasurable gave him a sense of the Infinite, and later of a Supreme Power that rules over all other powers.

Other important psychological factors in religion are fear[1] and curiosity. Primitive man found 'the unknown and the extraordinary to be disturbing epiphanies'.[2] Unusual things, situations and persons were felt to be possessed of some curious quality which aroused ambivalent emotions of terror and fascination. Such experiences bring man to his knees. This means that man's experiences of the *Numinosum* play a fundamental part in primitive religion and that these experiences have been and continue to be common to all forms of religion.

[1] 'The life of a primitive man can be compared with the progress of somebody walking through a modern electricity works with its engines and high tension cables. Everywhere he finds warnings saying "Do not touch", "Danger of Death".' Max Haller: *Die primitiven Religionen*: quoted by Oskar Pfister: *Christianity and Fear* (1948) p. 151.

[2] Mircea Eliade: *Patterns in Comparative Religion* (1958) pp. 7 ff.

Chapter IV

RELIGION AND PSYCHOLOGICAL CONCEPTS

In this chapter we are concerned to consider some of those psychological concepts which are of great importance for the study of religion, and we begin with instincts and the general concept of the unconscious, since much that distinguishes the religious life has its origin in the activity of the instincts operating below the level of ordinary everyday awareness.

Instincts

Instincts have been defined in various ways. William James defined them as 'the faculty of acting in such a way as to produce certain ends without foresight of the end, and without previous education in the performance'.[1] If this definition be compared with one provided by William McDougall who said that an instinct is

> an innate disposition which determines the organism to perceive (to pay attention to) any object of a certain class, and to experience in its presence a certain emotional excitement and an impulse to action which finds expression in a specific mode of behaviour in relation to that object[2]

we perceive that there is a considerable difference in the scope and nature of instincts. Stout comments that

> the history of thought concerning instinct, subsequent to Darwin, embraces two broadly contrasted tendencies. On the one hand there has been the attempt to render the concept strictly biological, and on the other there has been the tendency to re-express the facts in psychological terms and to explore the mental characteristics of instinctive process. . . .[3]

[1] James: *Principles of Psychology* (1901) Vol. II. p. 383.
[2] McDougall: *Outline of Psychology* (1923) p. 110.
[3] Stout: *Manual of Psychology*: 4th edn. 12th impression: revised C. A. Mace (1932) p. 332.

It is a common criterion of instinct that it results in the performance of actions which are perfectly performed from the outset, and prior to all experience or practice; but if this is accepted as the criterion of instinct it will hardly apply beyond the realm of the insect and lower animal kingdom. Instinctive behaviour for man is essentially conditioned by intelligent consciousness. Whatever innate dispositions a child is born with, among them is the capacity to learn by experience: 'there is every reason to believe that the purest instinctive action is the outcome of a distinctly mental process' [1] and that this mental process involves (as do all mental processes) three factors, the cognitive, affective and conative.

Religious Sentiment

Every instinct is associated with a specific emotion, an association of particular importance, as we shall see when we come to discuss worship and man's experience of the numinous. For example, the instinct of flight, which is associated with the perception of danger, gives rise to the emotion of fear; the parental instinct to tender feeling; the instinct of curiosity to the emotion of wonder, and the instinct of submission to negative self-feeling. Many of these emotions form an emotional complex. The emotion of admiration, for instance, is a complex emotional state which implies the pleasurable perception of an object or situation involving the emotion of wonder and negative self-feeling (from the instinct of self-abasement). If admiration is blended with the emotion of fear, it gives rise to yet another affective complex, awe. If gratitude be added to this complex of awe then we have another basic religious emotion – reverence. The reason why reverence is the deepest of all emotions is that there are comparatively few, if any, non-religious situations or personalities capable of evoking such a highly affective complex of wonder, fear, gratitude and negative self-feeling. These particular emotional reactions are fundamental to man's religious experiences and form the 'master sentiment' of religion. This master sentiment completes that 'hierarchy of purposes, attitudes and emotions in which relatively narrow and immediate aims and values are subordinated to others which are wider and more permanently valid'.[2] The assumption behind this statement

[1] McDougall: *Social Psychology* (1928) pp. 20 ff.
[2] Margaret Phillips: *The Education of the Emotions through Sentiment Development* (1937) p. 261.

is that there is some supreme value or Object about which the whole range of human emotions may finally be organized. But

> to apprehend, love and respond to the whole of reality is obviously, for finite minds, a task which can never be fully achieved. To apprehend, love and respond to a part, aspect or symbol is easier. Hence there is always the possibility that approach along any line may be arrested before the 'whole' is reached, and that there will then come into existence 'pseudo-religious' emotions and attitudes, taking as their real objects, parts or symbols, which emotions and attitudes are, however, only with difficulty to be distinguished from the true religious sentiment.[1]

The argument that the religious sentiment is the completion of a hierarchy of sentiments, has its counterpart in Dr Hadfield's 'Law of Completeness'.[2]

> Every organism is impelled to move towards its own completeness. Fullness of life is the goal of life; the urge to completeness is the most compelling motive of life. . . . As nature abhors a vacuum so every organism abhors incompleteness. In religion the craving for completeness and the sense of incompleteness is well marked; indeed, it appears to be the basis of religion. Before the terrible thud of the cyclone the South Sea savage is awakened by the feeling of his own weakness and insufficiency, and falls down in worship before the power which moves the hurricane to his destruction. Did we feel no sense of incompleteness we should have no 'fear' of God, no need of God, no love for God. . . . Psychologically the urge to completeness is most clearly marked in the instincts. Every instinct actively craves expression.[3]

This instinctual craving for completeness is in agreement with McDougall's 'hormic' interpretation of the instincts. McDougall uses the word *hormé* to describe the fact that instinct in man always seeks expression in some form of purposeful activity, that all his activities, even his dreams and psycho-pathological symptoms, exhibit some urge to reach a goal, however ill-defined that goal may actually be, in consciousness. Man's instinctual urge for completeness is basic to religion; man has a craving for God, though his realization of what that End is has varied greatly from age to age. It is this fact that caused Jung to define religion as 'the fruit and culmination of the completeness of life'.[4]

[1] Margaret Phillips: op. cit. p. 263.
[2] See J. A. Hadfield: *Psychology and Morals* (1925) chap. VIII.
[3] J. A. Hadfield: op. cit. pp. 61–2.
[4] Jung: *Psychology and Religion: West and East*: Collected Works. Vol. 11 (1958) p. 42.

Instinct and Religion

Some psychologists have suggested that among his many instincts man has a specifically religious instinct, but this is to advance too simple a psychological explanation for the existence of what is obviously a highly complex activity. The religious life involves the active collaboration of several instincts including those which relate to man's gregarious and sexual nature.

The gregarious instinct as it operates in human society makes the individual sensitive not only to the influence of group suggestion but also to the fear of being separated from his fellow men. Furthermore, the influence of society tends to modify the instinctual behaviour of the individual in a way that gives rise to what Freud called the Superego. These modifications operate in such a way that the energies of the crude instincts are directed to higher and more varied objectives. This process which is known as sublimation operates strongly in connexion with man's sexual instinct.

Some writers have held that religion is 'nothing-but' an expression of the sex instinct. Such a view arises from a rather inadequate appreciation of the nature of religion and from a too restricted view of sex. It overlooks the fact that the sex instinct plays a prominent part in most forms of human activity, but it is not so much the sexual energies themselves that are important as the ends to which they are devoted. 'True piety is earthly love transcendentalised, and the saint is the lover, purified, refined and perfected.' [1] Sex is one of the highest as well as one of the crudest of all forms of human interest. It is natural that since religion relates to the whole of a man's life and not to some rarified part of it, that religion should be related to man's sexual life. Starbuck showed that conversions occurring during adolescence are accompanied by emotions which are clearly related to the subject's developing sexual life. Furthermore, it is natural that situations in religion involving personal contacts between the human self and the Other (Buber's I–Thou relationship) should be described in the language of love and sexual relationships. As we shall have occasion to see later on, the symbolical language of mysticism is in large measure derived from the activities of the unconscious which, being strongly instinctual by nature, furnishes symbolical forms which are emotionally suited to experiences of a sublimated libidinal kind.

[1] G. Stanley Hall: *The Psychology of Adolescence*: Vol. II. p. 294.

The Unconscious

We have already seen that McDougall stressed the conative nature of instinct. This feature is of immediate relevance for our consideration of the unconscious because behind our day-to-day awareness there is 'a vast hormic organization of which a great part is never represented directly in consciousness, while, of the residue, much that has been once in consciousness, can never normally and in its own character reach the conscious level again'.[1] Certain aspects of our conscious life, such as the fact that each of us has a much larger volume of experience than is present in consciousness at any one time; the fact that 'forgotten' experiences suddenly engage our conscious attention and excite strong emotional responses; the fact that abnormal mental occurrences exercise a strong influence on our ordinary waking experience, call for some such psychological concept as the unconscious.[2] The unconscious seems to be a level of activity which is complementary and compensatory to our ordinary conscious life. It is both a deposit for discarded or repressed ideas and a creative treasury from which images and ideas emerge of a highly significant value. Psycho-analysis by the use of special techniques has been able to bring into consciousness experiences forgotten by the subject, techniques which have not only contributed to the relief of emotional conflicts but also have provided evidence that mental activities can and do operate outside consciousness.

Freud on the Unconscious

The position has been well expressed by Freud who says:

> To most people who have had a philosophical education the idea of anything mental which is not also conscious is so inconceivable that it seems to them absurd and refutable simply by logic. I believe this is only because they have never studied the mental phenomena of hypnosis and dreams, which – quite apart from pathological manifestations – necessitate this conclusion . . . an idea that is conscious now is no longer so a moment later on, although it can become so again under certain conditions that are easily brought about. What an idea was in the interval we do not know. We can say that it was *latent* and by this mean that it was

---

[1] T. P. Nunn: *Education: Its Data and First Principles* (1941) p. 62.

[2] 'We spend the greater part of our life in the unconscious; we sleep or daydream. . . . It is incontestable that in every important situation in life our consciousness is dependent upon the unconscious.' Jung: *Seminar: On Children's Dreams* (1938–1939) quoted Jolande Jacobi: *The Psychology of C. G. Jung* (1942) pp. 7–8.

> *capable of becoming conscious* at any time, or, if we say that it was *unconscious* we are giving an equally correct description. Thus 'unconscious' in this sense of the word coincides with 'latent and capable of becoming conscious'.[1]

The unconscious proper contains not only elements which have been 'forgotten' but also instinctual energies which have never been in consciousness.[2] These instinctual forces fall into two groups, the sexual and the egoistic. The unconscious is, therefore, a repository for all psychic processes which are not in consciousness and for those which cannot emerge into consciousness without overcoming certain 'resistances'. Repression operates in a three-fold manner: (1) it prevents unconscious elements from entering consciousness and is itself the result of early social training exerted upon the infantile mind by the conventions and moral standards of society; (2) it opposes attempts aimed at investigating the contents of the unconscious; (3) it is a dynamic barrier which functions as a *censor* to those mental events which seek to appear in consciousness. The censor is not always active, and when relaxed certain unconscious elements appear as in dreams.

Because of its instinctual character, the unconscious for Freud is thought of as being predominantly sexual in character but it should be noted that

> Freud does not only employ the expression 'sexuality' in the ordinary sense as 'the sum of those physical and psychical phenomena which refer to the propagation of the species, or the functions of the reproductive instinct and organs', but also in a much more extended sense, which coincides to all intents and purposes with the word 'love'.[3]

The unconscious comes into existence as the result of repression following an extended conflict between the child's innate instinctual endowment and the inhibiting conventions of the family and society. Jung agrees with Freud in recognizing that the unconscious comes into existence with the growth of the individual, but holds that in addition to the 'personal' unconscious there is an unconscious which is inborn and not due to repressive processes. Jung, therefore, places greater emphasis upon the hereditary aspect of the unconscious.

[1] Freud: *The Ego and the Id* (1935) pp. 10–11.
[2] See Freud: *Introductory Lectures on Psycho-Analysis* (1940) pp. 287 ff.
[3] Oskar Pfister: *Some Applications of Psycho-Analysis* (1923) p. 52.

Jung on the Unconscious

Jung's concept may be approached by way of analogy. H. G. Baynes, in the translator's preface to Jung's *Psychological Types* (1938), says: 'the lungs of the new-born infant know how to breathe, the heart knows how to beat, the whole co-ordinated organic system knows how to function, only because the infant's body is the product of inherited functional experience'. The 'knowing-how' of the child's body represents the whole phylogenetic history of man: if, therefore, there is a functional inheritance in the physical organism why should not man's psychical inheritance also be phylogenetic? It is this type of argument that caused Jung to promulgate the concept of a *racial* or *collective* unconscious common to and inherited by all men. 'Man is born with a brain that is the result of development in an endlessly long chain of ancestors.' [1] The collective unconscious[2] contains the psychical tendencies and dispositions common to the whole race, it is

> the all-controlling deposit of ancestral experience from untold millions of years, the echo of prehistoric world events to which every century adds an infinitesimally small amount of variation and differentiation. . . . It seems in its totality a sort of timeless world-image with a certain aspect of eternity opposed to our momentary conscious image of the world.[3]

Knowledge of the contents of the collective unconscious has been made possible, according to Jung, by comparing the mythological patterns of various religions with the complexes and dream symbolisms collected from many sources. The manner in which the collective unconscious produces the primordial symbolism of mankind will be discussed in the next chapter; what we have now to discuss is the nature of the psychical energy – libido – which is the potential of all human activities.

Libido

Psycho-analytically libido is the name given to the dynamic aspect of sexual instincts, but more generally it refers to the energy which operates in all psychical processes. Libido may be likened to the waters of a stream which by being diverted into certain channels can

[1] Jung: *Contributions to Analytical Psychology* (1928) p. 156.

[2] 'Jung has more recently employed an alternative term [for the collective unconscious], the "objective Psyche", thus expressing his view that the psyche is just as much an object as the world of outer fact.' See Michael Fordham: *The Objective Psyche* (1958) pp. 32 ff.

[3] Jung: *Contributions to Analytical Psychology* (1928) p. 162.

be raised to higher levels to give an increase in potential. Such a process is generally referred to as 'transformation' or 'sublimation'. Thus, for Freud, all the higher activities of man are the result of sublimations of the sexual instincts. Jung's definition of libido is an amplified version of the Freudian concept. Jung does not deny that many expressions of libidinal energy are intimately related to sexual activities, but he holds that as man in the course of his evolution extended the range of his interests so his libidinal energy was diverted from its primary sexual expression to objectives largely desexualized. In situations described as religious or numinous libido presents man's reactions in terms of primordial symbols. Jung expresses this view as follows: 'The psychological machine which transforms energy [libido] is the symbol. . . .' [1] 'The transformation of libido through the symbol is a process that has been taking place since the beginning of time and its effectiveness continues.' [2] This raises the question why man at early levels of culture wished to transform his libido to some analogue which gave a symbolical rather than a direct satisfaction? Jung concludes that it was because man found that by desexualizing libido he could release energy that would be available for other and higher interests. It may be suggested that these 'higher interests' are those by which man hopes to achieve that completeness of life which Dr Hadfield described as 'the basis of religion'. Desexualized libido is that supply of energy by which man has produced the whole range of activities which together make up civilization and express his reactions to the mystery of life and death.

Libido and History

Libido manifests itself in ways that are often the subject-matter of human history. It incites man to new and creative activities and also permits him to sink into long periods of seemingly uncreative inertia. The regressive tendency of the libido is the psychological expression of man's desire to return to the Mother – a tendency which Freud and Jung explained in different ways. Anthropologically it appears that this recessive phenomenon is a cardinal phase in human history, associating itself with that fatigue of the primitive mind which lends itself to an uncritical acceptance of what is communicated within the tribe. But this 'inertia of pause' is a highly significant factor in the creative development of man. In much the same way as there is an accumulation of psychic energy when some obstacle is encountered

[1] Jung: op. cit. p. 50. [2] ibid. p. 54.

in an individual's life, so there are periods when the race, or some part of it, 'pauses' until this accumulation results in some new and sometimes highly original development. That these processes cover long periods of history in no way invalidates the parallel.

> There are epochs in the history of civilization which are particularly characterized by a storing of the libido in the sense that from the reservoir of mythological and religious thought forms, new adaptations to the real processes and data are made. A significant example is the Renaissance, which a study of renaissance literature and a visit to the renaissance cities, e.g., Florence, make evident in a high degree. . . .[1]

This means that the *programme* of the libido as exhibited in the activities of the personal psyche is also the *programme* of civilization. This parallel is of special importance for religion since it shows itself in particularly significant forms in world mythology. For instance, the familiar mythological pattern of the dragon-fight, with the victorious hero and *the bound maiden set free*, or the equally familiar pattern of Mother and Child, are vivid symbolizations of the reversal of a negative libido to a positive libido. Anthropologically it represents the movement from an old integration of custom to a new differentiation; psychologically it represents that process of Individuation which Jung says is the basic desire of all men; religiously it represents that re-orientation or conversion of personality whereby a man is released from the 'bondage of sin' into the 'glorious liberty of the sons of God'.

Introversion and Extraversion

These terms stand for two attitudes which distinguish the life of the individual psyche (and, according to some historians, certain periods of culture).

> Introversion or extraversion, as a typical attitude, means an essential bias which conditions the whole psychic process, establishes the habitual reactions, and thus determines not only the style of behaviour, but also the nature of subjective experience. And not only so, but it also denotes the kind of compensatory activity of the unconscious which we may expect to find.[2]

An introvert is a person who has an 'inward-looking' attitude to life, while the extravert has an 'outward-looking' attitude. In the same

[1] Silberer: *Problems of Mysticism and Symbolism* (1917) pp. 305–6; see also Jacob Burckhardt: *The Civilization of the Renaissance* (Eng. trans. 1944).

[2] Jung: *Modern Man in Search of a Soul* (1936) p. 99.

way as the unconscious stands in a compensatory relationship to consciousness, so introversion and extraversion are compensatory attitudes. If a man is an introvert in his conscious life, then in his unconscious he is an extravert, and vice versa. Although all men have a dominant attitude, no one person is a complete extravert or a complete introvert, most people are not only a mixture of both, but their attitudinal habitus may change at different times in their personal lives. Each of these attitudes is related by Jung to one of four functions, thought, feeling, intuition and sensation. So that an introvert or an extravert may be characterized by any one of these four types.

In addition to the personal aspects of Introversion and Extraversion, it has been argued that certain ages exhibit one or other of these two attitudes, e.g. the Middle Ages appear as introverted when compared with the Renaissance or the modern world. This statement is not to be regarded as a value judgement, since each attitude stands in a complementary relationship to the other. In something of the same way as 'normality' is achieved by individuals who recognize the compensatory nature of their functional attitudes, so the reconciliation of opposites within an extended historical context constitutes one of the main themes of religious and historical movements. The Yin-Yang of the Chinese, the personification of *Rta* in the *Rig Veda*, the principle of the unification of opposites, the existence of Mitra and Varuna, the two guardians in Hindu mythology, and the concept of Tao, each represents, as does the Christian opposition of God and the Devil, a metaphysical example of the complementariness of opposed attitudes.

Anima and *Animus*

When a man becomes aware of the unrealized potentialities of his psyche, he discovers within the unconscious his own soul-image. In the male this image is feminine in character – *anima*; in the female it is masculine in character – *animus*. The relevance of this distinction for the symbolical expression of the unconscious needs no lengthy explanation. That a man sees his soul as a female figure is evidenced in dreams and in the mythological themes of world religions where it appears as a *leit-motif*, in such familiar forms as the moon-goddess, and in the various images of the *Magna Mater*.

Projection

As a psychological mechanism, projection is intimately connected with the concept of the Complex.[1] Complexes, which appear to enjoy an autonomous existence within the unconscious, 'project' themselves on to external things. A great deal of the mythology of religion is the result of the projection of automonous complexes on to situations expressive of a whole range of motifs such as Life and Death, Re-birth and Resurrection, themes which are as fundamental to historical religions as they are to mystery cults. The fact that these autonomous complexes are often projected on to particular situations and personalities provides one explanation of the multitudes of gods which populate polytheistic religions.

Complex and Oedipus Complex

The word 'complex' is generally taken to mean 'an associated group of ideas, partly or wholly repressed, strongly tinged with emotion, and in conflict with other ideas or groups of ideas more or less accepted by the individual.'[2] The recall of any one of the constituent elements brings the whole complex into consciousness together with its emotional associations. If at any time a complex should occupy the whole psychic field of an individual who is in a highly emotional condition, the individual would appear to be 'possessed' by the complex. There are, of course, complexes which are common to everyone. The child, for instance, collects a mass of memories, emotions and ideas around his father and mother, and these give rise to the father-complex and the mother-complex, or as they are sometimes called, when the emphasis is upon fatherhood or motherhood rather than upon a particular person – *an imago.*[3] According to Freud the first of these two particular complexes is the more important, because it is associated with the Oedipus Complex which Freud used in his explanation of the origin of religion.

The Oedipus Complex takes its name from the legend of Oedipus

[1] Complexes come into existence as the result of an emotional shock by which a part of the human personality is 'split off'. These split-off portions act as autonomous bodies in the sphere of consciousness and seem to possess their own 'voices' and appear as objective existences in external situations.

[2] J. Drever: *Dictionary of Psychology* (1958) p. 45.

[3] The idea of the complex was recognized in systems other than those of psychoanalysis; Herbart, for instance, postulated *apperception-masses* and William James described the *many selves* within the one personality.

son of Laios,[1] king of Thebes, who being exposed as an infant by his father's orders, returned as a man and, unaware of his royal parentage, slew a stranger who was his father and married unwittingly his own mother Jocasta. This legend is used by Freud to typify the boy's longing for his mother:

> At first it is the mother's breast which is the object of his desire, together with the other comforts and satisfactions, that she can provide for him, but later, as he develops, his desires become at first vaguely and then clearly sexual. Seeing in his father a hated rival, he longs to kill him in order to possess his mother. . . . On the other hand he can admire him and it is this combination of hatred, fear and admiration which results in identification with him; he 'becomes' his father, and so in a symbolical way can possess his mother . . . it is an unconscious, not conscious, solution.[2]

The Oedipus Complex is, therefore, characterized by a certain ambivalence involving hatred and affection for the one and the same parent, and, since our unconscious life is intimately connected with our infantile emotions, it is easy to understand why opposed affective elements, which co-exist easily in the mind of the child, exhibit a similar opposition in the adult mind. Freud claimed that the Oedipus Complex is universal, but this statement needs qualifying in two ways. Anthropologically it is not at all clear how this could apply to societies which are not patriarchal in structure. On the psychological side it is possible that every male is the subject of this complex, but there is no evidence that it is active in everybody.[3] This is substantially the position set out by Charles Baudouin:

> The Oedipus Complex is of very frequent occurrence . . . yet it would be false to maintain that the majority of men are in fact or by desire either incestuous or parricidal. The affair is much simpler. These impulses must be classed among the palaeolithic monsters . . . vestiges from very early childhood dating from a period of life when the child is absolutely amoral; vestiges which have to be thrust into the subconscious at the first onset of 'the moral age'.[4]

---

[1] A most interesting discussion of the *Laios-complex* is to be found in Ian Suttie: *Origins of Love and Hate* (1939) pp. 127 ff. Suttie draws an important distinction between patriarchal and matriarchal systems of society, saying that: 'We find a systematic difference in myth, theology, ritual and sacrifice, ethics and other mental characters between matriarchal and patriarchal peoples, which seems to me to indicate that the two cultures respectively derive their inspiration from and appeal to different levels of psychic development' (op. cit. p. 133).

[2] Michael Fordham: *The Life of Childhood* (1944) p. 20.

[3] W. H. R. Rivers: *Conflict and Dream* (1932) p. 144 f.

[4] Charles Baudouin: *Psycho-Analysis and Aesthetics* (1924) p. 205.

The relegation of this complex to the status of a vestigial psychic process does not necessarily disprove the widespreadness of its operation, for there is substantial evidence that this complex appears among peoples and cultures different from those of the civilized West. Sachs, for instance, writes that 'the situation which occurs in *Hamlet* is common to all humanity, and this is the primary reason why Shakespeare's tragedy appeals to men of all races and nations . . .' [1] and proceeds to draw a parallel between a negro John, who was the son of the chief witch-doctor, and Hamlet's own royal position. The father in both cases dies mysteriously, and John the negro dreams that he sleeps with his mother. Sachs offers other examples of a similar kind so that it seems that the Oedipus Complex operates at many levels and in many cultures, but what is not clear is how far it is to be treated as 'real' or how far it is symbolical of something else.

For Freud, as we have seen, the Oedipus Complex was a 'possession complex' in which the boy regarded his mother as the source of sexual gratification: Jung regarded it as more in the nature of a symbolical expression of the desire for re-birth, 'as a regressive product of the revival of the archaic modes of the function, outweighing actuality'.[2] This regressive activity of the libido is related by Jung to the process of *individuation* which is one of the most persistent desires of man's psychical life.

Individuation

In common with Lévy-Bruhl, Jung held that there was no trace of individuality in the psychology of primitive man who was more or less identified with the collective psyche. The emergence of the individual from this psychological collectivism is of primary importance for the development of mankind since it is the means whereby the self is born of the conflict between the world of collective consciousness and the world of individual awareness. This conflict is 'the old play of hammer and anvil: the suffering iron between them will in the end be shaped into an unbreakable whole – the individual'.[3] The achievement of personality is 'nothing less than the optimum development of the whole individual human being'.[4]

Individuation as a psychological process appears in religion as the

[1] W. Sachs: *Black Hamlet* (1937) p. 177.

[2] T. W. Mitchell: *Problems in Psycho-pathology*, quoted by H. Crichton-Miller: *Psycho-Analysis and its Derivatives* (1933) p. 191.

[3] Jung: *The Integration of the Personality* (1940) p. 27.

[4] Jung: *The Development of Personality*: Collected Works: Vol. 17. p. 171.

desire for re-birth; it is not only one of the main incentives in the life of the individual, it is also one of the main engagements of religion. It is that craving for completeness which, whether it be described as 'man's essential quest' or as the desire 'for union with the Other', is the *telos* of all religious activity. When in ordinary life a man tries to establish a place for himself in society he has to come to terms with the external world. The nature and the result of this struggle will to a large extent depend upon his particular psychological 'type', but when he has achieved some degree of social 'establishment' he may become aware of aspects of his interior life which were suppressed or ignored in his earlier years. This inner life now demands his attention so that the individual is confronted with the difficult problem of resolving oppositions within his psyche and within the universe (for man is by nature metaphysically curious), problems of Good and Evil, Light and Darkness, Life and Death. If he is by habit or training a religious man he will find some symbolical tradition that will help him to resolve these oppositions. If not, the process will involve much interior suffering before he is able to be delivered from the burden of these oppositions and is re-born a 'new man'. Hence St Paul's expression 'a new man in Christ'. Religion, in so far as it is something more than a statement of belief, enables a man to reconcile aspects of his inner and outer life which he has so far failed to accomplish by his own efforts, and thus to achieve a complete and balanced personality.[1]

* * *

In this chapter we have considered some of those concepts which are most relevant to the psychology of man as a religious being. Man is a creature whose life is rooted in the psychological and social heritage of the race, but whose activities are strongly influenced by the *hormic*, prospective-seeking nature of the libido. Whatever beliefs may be entertained about the nature of that Object to which man both consciously and unconsciously directs his life, we need to ask ourselves how objects or situations described as numinous or sacred

[1] 'Among all my patients in the second half of life – that is to say, over thirty-five – there has not been one whose problem in the last resort was not that of finding a religious outlook on life. It is safe to say that every one of them fell ill because he had lost that which the living religions of every age have given to their followers, and none of them has been really healed who did not regain his religious outlook. This of course has nothing whatever to do with a particular creed or membership of a church.' Jung: *Modern Man in Search of a Soul* (1936) p. 264: Collected Works: Vol. 11. p. 334.

come to be invested with a highly significant range of symbols, many of which seem to be common to religion at all levels. Analytical Psychology advances arguments which explain such a process as being due to the operation of certain functional powers within the collective unconscious. These symbolical forms are said to be the means by which man's perception of the Ineffable becomes at one and the same time psychologically expressible and psychically satisfying. If this is so, it is important that we should consider these explanations.

Chapter V

ARCHETYPES, SYMBOLS, MYTHS

Religion claims the 'whole' man and, therefore, includes all sides of existence, those which are capable of being apprehended by reason, perceived through the senses, responded to by the emotions and intuited immediately without rational consideration. Since religion by its very nature refers to both the transcendent and immanent aspects of that mystery which pervades the universe and the life of man, it cannot be exhaustively described in rational language. Yet man for an incalculable length of time has possessed a 'language' which enables him to express his sense of the 'sacred' in a way that no other language can – the medium of symbols and primordial imagery.

Archetypes

The concept of Archetypes is one of Jung's most important contributions to the psychology of religion; but because Jung has described this concept in such a variety of ways[1] it may perhaps be more helpful to describe (rather than to define) this concept in terms of the way in which it is said to operate. The collective unconscious (objective psyche) contains instincts which not only influence the way man behaves, thinks and feels, but also provides a range of symbolic images which enable man to express his reactions to situations and experiences which by their very nature defeat all attempts to express them intellectually. The means whereby instinctual energy (libido in a generalized sense) produces this 'currency' of significant images are the archetypes proper. Archetypes are 'dominants' which, operating within the collective unconscious, 'create' those symbolic patterns by which man expresses his reactions to the numinous and the mysterious. The manner in which these dominants operate has been compared to the 'lattices' in crystalline substances. Every class of crystal is distinguished by the number of facets and the angle at

[1] See Jolande Jacobi: *Psychological Reflections – An Anthology of the Writings of C. G. Jung* (1953), and Jolande Jacobi: *Complex, Archetype, Symbol* (1959).

which these facets are inclined to each other. If a quantity of crystals of the same kind be dissolved they will, when the solution has been evaporated, reappear possessed of the same crystalline structure as before because of the operation of their particular lattice. The lattice is a non-material function which determines the actual structure of crystalline substances. Similarly archetypes are the 'lattices' or dominants operating within the 'waters' of the collective unconscious, producing significant patterns, or psychical 'crystallizations' which appear in dreams and consciousness as *primordial images* and symbols.

The word archetype is used in two senses, (*a*) as the name for dominants or processes within the collective unconscious, and (*b*) as an adjective to qualify imagery produced by these dominants. The chief characteristics of archetypal images are that they are archaic, non-personal, unconscious in origin and common to all races and all times. They are the means of expressing psychologically the significance of situations whose rational counterparts appear less vividly and less satisfactorily as dogmas and doctrines. Of Jung's many definitions of archetypes proper the following is one of the most illuminating:

> Inasmuch as the child comes into the world with a differentiated brain, predetermined by heredity and therefore also individualized, its reactions to outside sense stimuli are not just any reactions but are specific, as a particular (individual) selection and form of apperception necessarily involves. These faculties can be proved to be inherited instincts and even preformations conditioned by the family. The latter are the *a priori*, formal conditions of apperception based on instincts. They set their anthropomorphic stamp upon the world of the child and of the dreamer. They are the archetypes, which blaze a definite trail for all imagination and produce astonishing mythological parallels in the images of a child's dreams and in the schizophrenic's delusions and even to a lesser degree in the dreams of both normal and neurotic persons. It is not a question of inherited ideas but of inherited possibilities for these.[1]

Of primordial imagery (archetypal imagery) the following definition is one of the most helpful:

> I term the image *primordial* when it possesses an archaic character. I speak of its archaic character when the image is in striking union with familiar mythological motives. In this case it expresses material primarily derived from the collective unconscious, while, at the same

[1] Jung: quoted in Jacobi: *Psychological Reflections* (1953) p. 36.

time, it indicates that the momentary conscious situation is influenced not so much from the side of the personal as from the collective. . . .

The primordial image (elsewhere also termed the 'archetype') is always collective, i.e., it is at least common to entire nations or epochs. In all probability the most important mythological motives are common to all times and races.[1]

Having discussed the difference between archetypes as functional dominants within the collective unconscious and archetypes as primordial images we can now consider the psychological nature of Symbols.

Symbols

Symbols like archetypal imagery are unconscious and instinctual by origin, they cannot be consciously invented and they must be distinguished from rationally composed *signs*. Symbols have played and continue to play a more prominent part in the religions of mankind than ideas. A. N. Whitehead has a profound remark on this matter of ideas versus symbols: 'it is characteristic of the learned mind to exalt words. Yet mothers can ponder many things which their lips cannot express. These many things which are thus known constitute the ultimate religious evidence beyond which there is no appeal.'[2] The things which the lips cannot express are among those situations which symbols are capable of expressing.

Freud and Jung both agreed that symbols are the product of instinctual activities within the unconscious, but they differed as to the method by which symbols are to be interpreted, particularly those symbols which appear in dreams. Freud interpreted dream-symbols (which he regarded as the 'royal road' into the unconscious) on a strictly causal principle; Jung, while employing this principle to some extent, included a *prospective* principle saying that some dreams were capable of being understood only in terms of the psyche's aim or *telos*. This agrees with what we have already said about the prospective aspect of man's psychical nature. Man is not completely dominated by his past; his activities, especially those which are expressed symbolically, must also be interpreted prospectively. It is this fact that makes symbolism such an important factor in religion.

When dealing with Individuation we said that 'the desire for rebirth is not only one of the main incentives in the life of the individual, it is also one of the main engagements of religion'. This is

[1] Jung: *Psychological Types* (1938) pp. 555–6.
[2] A. N. Whitehead: *Religion in the Making* (1926) p. 67.

F

clearly to be seen in those symbols which are concerned with this particular desire:

> The symbol always says: In some such form as this will a new manifestation of life, a deliverance from the bondage and weariness of life be found. The libido which is freed from the unconscious by means of the symbol is symbolised as a young or rejuvenated god . . . the motif of the God-renewal is universal and, therefore, presumably familiar.[1]

This motif is expressed in such myths as those of the hero emerging from the interior of the great Monster of the Deep, what Frobenius called 'the universal hatching-out'. Myths and symbols expressing 're-birth' present the individual with intimations of relief from the frustrations of spiritual (psychological) death. This is the reason why in all religions symbols that express themes of salvation, re-birth and new life play such a prominent part. They are a symbolical assurance of man's trust that he can be delivered out of 'the body of this death'.

Symbols and Society

An inherited symbolism is itself part of that tradition which helps to maintain the structure of society, but different epochs of civilization disclose different attitudes towards symbolism. A symbol is the expression of some theme that cannot be expressed in any other or better way. But if this theme should 'evaporate' then a symbol becomes 'dead', and as such can be said to retain only a historical significance. We may take H. O. Taylor's statement that the symbolism which dominated the life of the Middle Ages was of a different type from that which characterized the life of the Renaissance.[2] During the Renaissance medieval symbolism was largely discounted not because it had ceased to express unconscious processes but because the 'symbolic attitude' of the age had changed. In the Middle Ages men tended to take an introverted attitude to existence, concentrating on the 'inner' life and the fact of death. It is significant that in the second half of the Middle Ages the word *macabre* appeared in France and, thereafter, life was described in terms of the Dance of Death. But during the Renaissance man's attention was directed outwards, and man lived as if his chief objective was to secure a monumental place in the annals of history.

Today another change of 'symbolic attitude' is taking place. In the same way as the complex social changes of the fifteenth and six-

[1] Jung: op. cit. p. 320.
[2] H. O. Taylor: *The Mediaeval Mind* (1930) 2 vols.

teenth centuries radically affected the Western attitude to the inherited symbolism of the Middle Ages, so today the sweeping social changes of mass industrialization are similarly affecting the symbolic attitude of peoples and individuals alike. Dr F. W. Dillistone, discussing these changes, asks: 'Can the distinctively Christian symbols, therefore, closely associated as they are with the environments out of which they originally emerged, survive in the altogether changed environment of the mid-twentieth century?' [1] The answer is that although the psychical nature of man, despite the scientific framework of his life, has not changed basically (and, indeed, cannot do so, so long as man remains man), yet because the symbolism of Western religion is still largely that of an introverted version of Christianity, it is incompatible with the extraverted interests of modern society and so the need is for some compensatory type of symbolism. Modern man requires a symbolism eloquent of human needs in a new social setting. This is imperative not only because symbols express human needs, but also because they promote social cohesion and carry certain psychological assurances without which man cannot continue to live. A society, or a religion, whose symbolism no longer appears meaningful is in danger of disintegrating or becoming obsolescent. The present existential view that 'God is dead' or the popular belief that Christianity is no longer relevant, is in reality an assertion that the symbols which express the God-idea (or what Jung calls the *God-imago*) have ceased to be meaningful. This is a change of symbolic attitude, not a denial of the spiritual truth which is enshrined in the word-symbol 'God' or the fundamental nature of Christianity. What is dead is not 'God' but the God-symbol, that is, it has for the time lost its contemporary appeal. This agrees with something which Jung said about archetypes. As we shall see a little later, the God-archetype is the means whereby man is able to 'know' God. If this archetype for the time being appears to be less significant than it once was it is because as an archetype (*not* as a reality) it resembles the bed of a river. This can dry up because the water has deserted it, though it may return at any time. 'An archetype is something like an old watercourse along which the water of life flowed for a time, digging a deep channel for itself. The longer it flowed the deeper the channel, and the more likely it is that sooner or later the water will return.' [2] The psychical waters of human life have for the time been

[1] F. W. Dillistone: *Christianity and Symbolism* (1955) p. 291.
[2] Jung, quoted in Jolande Jacobi: *Psychological Reflections* (1953) p. 36.

diverted into other channels, but man's sense of isolation, frustration, pessimism, and preoccupation with world annihilation are undeniable evidence of his need for a re-animated symbolism that will carry that assurance of completion, unity, harmony and purpose which the *God-imago* has hitherto conveyed, and conveyed in a manner which no purely intellectual statement has ever been able to do. Symbols arising from the collective unconscious of mankind have been and are the means whereby the transcendental makes itself convincingly present in human experience.[1]

Symbolism and Historical Religions

Historical religions begin with traditions which they inherit from the past.[2] Every genuine religious tradition, since it is expressive of man's psychical needs and experiences, is a form of collective symbolization whose 'shape' is conditioned by historical circumstances. But this form of collective symbolism, when it is concerned with a religion which has at its centre a historic Figure, is a symbolism controlled by the framework of fact and institution. The historic Figure himself becomes a symbol of man's needs and aspirations and is, at the same time, expressive of that element of reality which stimulates the creative activities of the objective psyche to promote a relevant series of primordial images. 'No great thing', says Jung, 'ever came into being without first being expressed in phantasy.'[3] This means that religions exist in symbolic forms long before they exist as historical traditions.

The traditions of Christianity embody a much wider volume of psychical facts than those which are labelled 'historical facts'. The historical facts of Christianity assume an additional significance because they are supported by those psychical *motifs* which have animated man's unconscious life from very early times, and also

[1] Cassirer – approaching this question of symbols from what may be called the philosophical aspect of philology – says that we must see in symbols 'an original way and tendency of expression which is more than a mere record of something initially given in fixed categories of real existence'. Symbols in myth, art and language are not imitations but *organs* of reality by means of which anything that is real discloses its true significance. See Ernst Cassirer: op. cit. p. 8.

[2] Buddhism adopted a substantial part of the Hindu tradition by a process of conventionalization and assimilation; Christianity took over the traditions of Old Testament and Hellenistic Judaism; Muhammadanism was heavily indebted to the traditions of Jewish, Zoroastrian and Christian monotheism. See R. H. Thouless: *Conventionalisation and Assimilation in Religious Movements* (1940). Appendix III.

[3] *Psychological Types* (1938) pp. 75–6.

because they themselves confer a certain 'historicity' on the psychological testimony of human experience. Such nature myths as those of Osiris, Marduk and Adonis are invested with a new significance when they are viewed in the light of the historical Jesus who is the 'verification' of the all-pervading pattern of the Dying-and-Rising-God who is the saviour of the world. Historical truths in religion exercise their power over believers not on rational grounds alone, but also because they verify that element of reality which is inherent in the archetypal imagery of the objective psyche. In other words, our conscious acceptance of such beliefs depends as much upon their connexion with the psychological past as it does upon historical evidence, faith and rational argument; Man expressed his apprehension of reality by primordial imagery ages before the theologian and the philosopher began their reasoned expositions and commentaries.

Myth

Before we consider myth as a psychological 'fact' it will be helpful to look at it in non-psychological contexts. Plato, for instance, used myth as the name for popular forms of explanation in much the same way as the New Testament employs the parable. But this is not how it is used by students of comparative religion. One of the best explanations is that given by Professor S. H. Hooke in *Myth and Ritual*[1] who shows that 'myth' and 'ritual' were invariably associated in the early cultures of the Eastern Mediterranean and Mesopotamian areas. Sir James Frazer, who defined mythology as the 'philosophy of primitive man', said that 'myths are documents of human thought in the embryo'.[2] We have devoted some space to discussing the nature of the 'primitive mind' and it is obvious that we cannot use the word 'primitive' to describe the rites and mythologies of Egypt and Mesopotamia. None the less in the myths of these highly developed civilizations there are threads which lead us to those primitive situations from which the myth-and-ritual pattern of ancient cultures is plainly derived.

Originally, says Professor Hooke, man's early preoccupations were with the 'practical' issues of life, with such problems as securing the rising and setting of the sun, the regular flooding of the Nile, with the

[1] S. H. Hooke: *Myth and Ritual – Essays on the Myth and Ritual of the Hebrews in Relation to the Culture Pattern of the Ancient East* (1933). See also A. M. Hocart: *Kingship* (1927); E. O. James: *Christian Myth and Ritual* (1937); S. H. Hooke: *The Labyrinth* (1935); Mircea Eliade: *Myths, Dreams and Mysteries* (1956).

[2] Frazer: *Myths of the Origin of Fire: An Essay* (1930).

physical well-being of the king, who in all these early cultures (and in many quite primitive communities) was the person upon whose health and virility the prosperity of the community was believed to depend.[1] In addition, there were the more personal problems of disease, luck and the uncertainty of the future, for which situations man devised rituals. These rituals have two elements, a point to which A. M. Hocart was the first to draw attention. These are 'the things done' (e.g. R. R. Marett's 'dancing-out' a problem or situation), and 'the things said'. The things done are the ritual proper, the things said are the myth. The myth is, therefore, the 'explanation' not only of *what* is actually being done in the rite itself, but also of *why* it is being done, that is, it is a description of some original situation out of which the ritual originally arose. To what extent such rituals were modelled by the archetypal processes of the objective psyche need not at the moment detain us.

Dr A. M. Blackman when dealing with the Egyptian Coronation Ritual in the Ramesseum Papyrus[2] shows that the spoken part of the ritual included the Osiris myth at considerable length, while C. J. Gadd in describing the Babylonian New Year Ritual,[3] in which Marduk was thought of as lying dead 'in the mountain', shows that the recitation of the Babylonian Creation myth, the *enuma elish* (to which the Hebrew Creation stories bear a close resemblance), is an essential part of the rite for securing the restoration of Marduk to life. Similar rituals existed in the religions of the early Greek, Minoan, Hittite, Elamite and Indus Valley civilizations. The close resemblances between them seem to indicate some degree of cultural borrowing, but whether this is so or not, it is clear that all such rituals and their accompanying myths are based primarily upon some original pattern which is the psychological expression of human needs and human reactions to particular situations. Ritual patterns such as the Sacred Marriage which refers to the union of the powers of fertility, and New Year Festivals which include stories of conflicts between such opponents as Horus and Set, Marduk and Tiamat, Yah-

[1] Frazer provides a wealth of evidence drawn from wide areas and many levels of civilization illustrating the fact that 'the motive for slaying a man-god is a fear lest with the enfeeblement of his body in sickness or old age his sacred spirit should suffer a corresponding decay, which might imperil the general course of Nature, and with it the existence of his worshippers, who believe the cosmic energies to be mysteriously knit up with those of their human divinity'. Frazer: *The Golden Bough* (abridged edn) chap. XXIV.

[2] See S. H. Hooke: *Myth and Ritual*, pp. 29 ff.

[3] op. cit. pp. 50 ff. and 61 ff.

weh and the Dragon, are all explicable on psychological grounds, since they clearly indicate man's reactions to physical regularities which in the course of experience were clothed in primordial imagery.

If it be asked 'why are such physical regularities clothed by the unconscious in phantasies *about* nature rather than in pictures *of* nature?' the answer is that the primitive mind did not draw the same philosophical distinction between the subjective and the objective aspects of life, but had an empathy with its surroundings (*participation mystique*) so that what happened outside man in a sense happened inside him. This explains why external events which were felt to be internal occurrences were clothed in primordial imagery. Furthermore, if it be asked 'why did primitive man think mythologically?' the answer is that situations thought of as being endowed with *mana* can be explained only by means which are not dominated by the principle of cause-and-effect.[1] Myths then may be looked upon as the epitomized reactions of man to that rationally inexplicable procession of need, crisis, calamity and creativity which characterizes human experience in all ages. Even today, despite the higher level of man's intellectual powers, there are recurring situations whose significance eludes rational explanation – life is a *drama* more mysterious than reason can elucidate or man can understand. It is for reasons of this kind that historical no less than non-historical religions have to express the highlights of existence in myth-and-ritual patterns.

But as soon as we have said this, we have to face the fact that the relationship between mythology and historical religion has been a matter of intellectual embarrassment to many theologians in the past, although a new appreciation of the nature of the myth is beginning to emerge among modern theologians. Professor Hooke in his Introduction to *The Labyrinth*[2] adds a significant note on the meaning of Myth. Explaining that the myth possesses a truth which is both 'wider and deeper than the narrow truth of history', Hooke goes on to say that

> an historical event can only take place once. From the historical point of view the battle of Waterloo is a single unique event which can never be repeated. But the essential truth of the myth lies in the fact that it embodies a situation of profound emotional significance, a situation,

---

[1] See Jung: *Contributions to Analytical Psychology* (1928) pp. 41–2, 112–13.

[2] *The Labyrinth – Further Studies in the Relation between Myth and Ritual in the Ancient World* (1935).

moreover, which is in its nature recurrent, and which calls for the repetition of the ritual which deals with the situation and satisfies the need evoked by it. . . .

Referring to Christianity as a new religion in the ancient world, Professor Hooke says that the appeal of the new religion

> lay not so much in the fact that it had its origin in historical events as in its *tremendum mysterium* of a dying and rising God, and of the ever-recurrent repetition in daily and yearly ritual of the central situation which had power to meet every kind of human need, not only to ensure eternal bliss, but to ensure the success of the homely activities of birth, marriage, fishing and harvest. It is in this sense that we may speak of the Christian myth, without the slightest reflection on the historical character of the events out of which the Christian religion sprang. The term is used to express the fact of the ever-recurring repetition of a situation in which human need is met by the life-giving potency of a sacral act.[1]

That the myth embodies a recurring situation of *profound emotional significance* is given a psychological explanation by Jung, who in his *Answer to Job*[2] discusses certain aspects of problems which he had dealt with earlier[3] in connexion with Christ both as a historical person and as a symbolical figure (*symbolum*). How are we, for instance, asks Jung, to interpret many of Christ's sayings, such as those from the Cross? Many commentators have failed to understand their real significance because they have declined to view them within a general mythical setting. 'If these sayings are detached from their mythical context, they can only be explained personalistically.'[4] If we interpret such a statement as 'I am the Way, and the Truth and the Life: no one comes to the Father but by me'[5] on strictly personalistic lines, we are likely, says Jung, to arrive at much the same conclusion as that reached by Jesus's own family, who took the mundane and severely humanistic view of most of his utterances, judging him to be 'beside himself'.

The dangerous limitations of purely personalistic types of interpretation caused Jung to ask 'What is the use of a religion without a mythos, since religion means, if anything at all, precisely that function which links us back to the eternal myth?'[6] But it is this use of the word *mythos* which engenders in many minds the suspicion that if we

[1] S. H. Hooke: op. cit. pp. ix, x.

[2] *Psychology and Religion: West and East*: Section VI. Collected Works: Vol. 11. pp. 356 ff.

[3] See *Aion*: Collected Works: Vol. 9. Section II.

[4] Jung: *Answer to Job* in Collected Works: Vol. 11. pp. 408 ff.

[5] John xiv. 6. [6] op. cit. p. 409.

view the doctrine of the Incarnation as a 'myth' then we are judging it to be 'untrue' – for many theologians in the past, and some in the present, have held that a myth is nothing more than a religious version of a fairy-tale. But mythology is not a series of elaborate fairy-tales, it is the psychologically created medium whereby transcendental reality (using these words in a theological sense) is given a 'this-worldly' objectivity. The *mythos* is the only way by which the Christian belief that Jesus is at one and the same time both fully God and fully man, can be satisfactorily presented.

> The fact that the life of Christ is largely myth does absolutely nothing to disprove its factual truth. Quite the contrary. I would even go so far as to say that the mythical character of a life is just what expresses its universal human validity. It is perfectly possible, for the unconscious or an archetype to take complete possession of a man and to determine his fate down to the smallest detail. At the same time objective, non-psychic parallel phenomena can occur which also represent the archetype. It not only seems so, it simply is so, that the archetype fulfils itself not only psychically in the individual, but objectively outside the individual. My own conjecture is . . . that the life of Christ is just what it had to be if it is the life of a god and a man at the same time.[1]

Theology, whatever its reactions to Jungian explanations, is unwise if it seeks to diminish the psychological value of the myth. Ian Henderson, discussing the value of Rudolf Bultmann's attempt to 'demythologize' the content of the New Testament[2] (a highly stimulating attempt whatever views individual readers may entertain about the soundness of his conclusions), quotes Theilicke as saying:

> The myth is a legitimate form of human thought: it is, in fact, the only one in which the supersensible can be grasped. There is no need to apologize for it, for just because it deals with the ultimate meaning of things, it attains to a dimension of depth, which scientific knowledge cannot reach.[3]

This is substantially the point of view of Paul Tillich: 'myth is more than a primitive world-view . . . it is the necessary and adequate expression of revelation'.[4] The form of the myth is determined both by the activity of the psyche and by the necessity of expressing the

[1] Jung: op. cit. p. 409.

[2] See Rudolf Bultmann: *Theology of the New Testament*: 2 vols. (1952, 1955), *Jesus Christ and Mythology* (1960).

[3] Ian Henderson: *Myth in the New Testament* (1952) pp. 50–1.

[4] See Paul Tillich: *The Protestant Era* (1951) pp. 18 ff., and *Systematic Theology* (1953) Vol. I. pp. 246 ff.

transcendental in a this-worldly manner. These two points would seem to explain why the mythological presentations of religion appear to vary but little from age to age.

Primordial Imagery, Art and Religion

Poets, artists and mystics have demonstrated down the ages that by the use of primordial images and symbols man is able to express his apprehension of a Power which both transcends and, at the same time, is immanent within the natural world and in man himself. These experiences defy logical description but poetry, art, drama, mime, ritual, liturgy, music and other creative arts are well fitted to describe the ineffable when they use archetypal imagery. This helps us to understand why Hegel ascribed such a high value to poetry as the medium for conveying man's apprehension of Spirit. The symbols which emerge from the objective psyche are highly charged with emotion because of their primordial origin, and provide mankind, at all levels of development, with the only available means of expressing that ambivalence of terror and love which is the result of an experience of Reality.

Gilbert Murray, comparing the tragedies of *Hamlet* and *Orestes*, refers to that continuity of thought-feeling which stirs modern no less than primitive man. Even in our highly lit and scientifically regulated world there are situations at which something within us

> leaps at the sight of them, a cry of the blood which tells us that we have known them always . . . a strange unanalysed vibration below the surface, an understanding of desires and fears and passions, long slumbering yet eternally familiar, which have for thousands of years lain near the root of our most intimate emotions and been wrought into the fabric of our most magical dreams.[1]

Beneath our modern life there moves a deep ancestral current which not only carries the experiences of the whole human race, but also enables us to respond to our apprehensions of the mystery of life in a way that no analytical or logical statement can. Nowhere is this more clearly to be seen than in religious art and worship, where the employment of ancestral forms and primordial imagery both captures and revives man's inherent sense of an eternal mystery.

[1] Gilbert Murray: '*Hamlet* and *Orestes*' in *The Classical Tradition in Poetry* (1927) pp. 238–40; cf. Maud Bodkin: *Archetypal Patterns in Poetry* (1934).

Chapter VI

FREUD ON RELIGION

Freud's attitude to religion is well expressed in two sentences near the end of his study of Leonardo da Vinci:

> Psycho-analysis has made us aware of the intimate connexion between the father-complex and the belief in God, and has taught us that the personal God is *psychologically* nothing other than a magnified father; it shows us every day how young people can lose their religious faith as soon as the father's authority collapses. We thus recognize the root of religious need as lying in the parental complex.[1]

Freud's studies of religion are all variations upon this theme of God the 'magnified father', but before we proceed to deal with these arguments we should look first into Freud's own religious background as this is admirably set out by Ernest Jones in his three-volume life of Freud. Ernest Jones says that we know two things about Freud's religious upbringing, first that he had a Catholic nannie in his first three years who took him with her to church; secondly, that although born of a Jewish family, it was a home with 'an almost entirely secular atmosphere'.[2] The usual religious experiences associated with adolescence seem not to have played any part in Freud's development, for he confessed that he had never had any belief in the existence of the 'supernatural'. Yet Freud was familiar from an early age with the Old Testament and later acquired a considerable knowledge of the New Testament and the religions of antiquity.

> Nevertheless, he went through his life from beginning to end as a natural atheist . . . that is to say, one who saw no reason for believing in the existence of any supernatural Being and who felt no emotional need for such a belief. The world of Nature seemed all-embracing and he could find no evidence of anything outside it.[3]

[1] Freud: *Leonardo da Vinci* (1932) p. 103.
[2] Ernest Jones: *Sigmund Freud* (1957) Vol. III. p. 375.
[3] Ernest Jones: op. cit. Vol. III. p. 376.

Freud himself frequently expressed surprise that intelligent people held religious beliefs, but what is not clear is why he himself as 'a natural atheist' should have been so deeply and so illuminatingly interested in the psychology of religion.

In Freud's view religion was the projection of the child's psychical relationship with its father. Even Jewish monotheism had behind it the nucleus of the father-figure, for once God was seen to be one, man could project more easily on to a single deity feelings which he had as a child directed towards his father. This view is directly related to Freud's belief that the mythologies of world religions show that religion itself is 'nothing other than psychological processes projected into the outer world'. Freud first published his arguments about the nature of religion in *Totem and Taboo* (1913) in which he attributed the origin not only of religion, but of civilization, morality, law and culture, to the psychological connexion between the Oedipus Complex and totemism as it existed within small primitive groups. Freud was especially indebted to Frazer's *Totemism and Exogamy* and *The Golden Bough* as well as to Robertson Smith's *Religion of the Semites*, which, he said, confirmed many ideas he had not previously dared to publish. From Frazer he learnt that the totem animal must not be killed except communally and that members of the same totemic group were not permitted to have sexual relations with women of the same tribe (hence, exogamy). These two practices were related by Freud to that situation to which he had given the name Oedipus Complex, a situation in which the son hates the father because of his own desire to possess his mother. As a result of these psychological associations Freud reached the conclusion that God was the projection of the father-figure, and that the sense of guilt, the practice of sacrifice, and standards of sexual morality within the tribe, were derived from the early forms of patriarchal totemism.

In subsequent works, Freud developed the ideas which he had discussed in *Totem and Taboo*. In *The Future of an Illusion* (1927) he defined religion (which was the 'illusion') as consisting of 'certain dogmas, assertions about facts and conditions of external (or internal) reality, which tell one something that one has not discovered oneself, and which claim that we should give them credence'.[1] It is significant that Freud's definition makes no reference whatever to experience, nor does it in any way refer to the fact that dogmas and statements of belief are based upon the richness of religious experiences. But

[1] op. cit. p. 43.

since religion is related 'to the most insistent wishes of mankind' – to man's desire to escape from the stern facts of reality – religion is nothing more than an expression of man's wishful thinking. This desire to escape from reality is related, for Freud, to the psychological factors which characterize the relations of a small boy to his father, a relationship which is strengthened by the child's vivid awareness of his helplessness in the face of the realities of the unknown world which confronts him. Man projects this infantile relationship on to the face of the external world, a world of cruelty, terror and stark indifference to human nature. It is, says Freud, difficult to believe that early man could have succeeded in facing the terrors of life had it not been for such comfort as was afforded by the illusion of religion.[1] If modern man would but employ his reason and thereby condition his emotions, he would be able to outgrow the childishness of an appeal to religion, an appeal that belongs properly to the childhood of the race. This argument was stated even more emphatically in *Civilization and its Discontents* (1930), where Freud said that 'the ordinary man cannot imagine [this] Providence in any other form but that of a greatly exalted father, for only such a one could understand the needs of the sons of men, or be softened by their prayers and placated by the signs of their remorse'.[2] By concentrating upon religion as a matter of paternally induced activities and by his singular omission of religion as experience, Freud was able to indicate a number of resemblances between religious observances and the behaviour of patients suffering from obsessive neuroses. It is true that a substantial part of religious observances is concerned with feelings of guilt, with the desire to find some means to control instinctual activities and with a highly conscientious attention to detail. Much the same psychical impulses distinguish the behaviour of neurotic personalities. But to describe the 'observances by means of which the faithful give expression to their piety . . . as a universal

[1] Freud's use of the word 'illusion' has been the subject of much criticism but Freud himself took care to point out that 'an illusion is not the same as an error, it is indeed not necessarily an error. Aristotle's belief that vermin are evolved out of dung, to which ignorant people still cling, was an error; . . . On the other hand, it was an illusion on the part of Columbus that he had discovered a new sea-route to India. The part played by his wish in this error is very clear. . . . It is characteristic of the illusion that it is derived from man's wishes. . . . Thus we call a belief an illusion when wish-fulfilment is a prominent factor in its motivation, while disregarding its relations to reality, just as the illusion itself does.' Freud: *The Future of an Illusion* (1934) pp. 53–4.

[2] op. cit. p. 23.

obsessional neurosis' is to overlook the fact that an obsessional neurosis is, so far as the individual patient is concerned, an abnormal and strictly personal activity, whereas religion is a universal and normal activity of mankind. Freud seems never to have considered the possibility that man might be by nature a 'religious animal'.

Several years later, Freud wrote his last book on religion and psychology, *Moses and Monotheism* (1939), which has largely been discounted because of the speculative nature of Freud's views and because leading Old Testament scholars have pointed to serious errors in Freud's argument, a matter to which we shall devote our attention a little later in this chapter.

Totem and Taboo

Since this book is the liveliest expression of Freud's views on religion, we must now consider it in some detail. In his introduction, Freud said that these four essays

> represent my first efforts to apply view points and results of psycho-analysis to unexplained problems of racial psychology . . .
>
> The two principal themes, totem and taboo . . . are not treated alike here. The investigation of totemism may be modestly expressed as: 'This is all that psycho-analytic study can contribute at present to the elucidation of the problem of totemism' . . . Totemism is a religio-social institution which is alien to our present feelings; it has long been abandoned and replaced by new forms. In the religions, morals and customs of the civilized races of to-day it has left only slight traces, and even among those races where it is still retained, it has had to undergo great changes. . . . In this book the attempt is ventured to find the original meaning of totemism through its infantile traces, that is, through the indications in which it reappears in the development of our own children.

Freud not only drew his anthropological material from many sources,[1] he also adopted the Darwinian theory as it had been elaborated by F. Atkinson who said that 'at a very early period man lived in small communities consisting of an adult male and a number of females and immature individuals, the males being driven off by the head of the group as soon as they became old enough to evoke his

[1] These sources included: J. F. M'Lennan: *Primitive Marriage* (1866) and an essay on 'The Worship of Animals and Plants'; W. Robertson Smith: *Animal Worship and Animal Tribes among the Arabs in the Old Testament* (1880); *The Religion of the Semites* (1889); Frazer: *Studies on Totemism* (1887); F. B. Jevons: *Introduction to the History of Religion* (1896); Spencer and Gillen: *The Beginnings of Religion and Totemism among the Australian Aborigines* (1905).

jealousy'.[1] Atkinson, who lived for many years in New Caledonia (in complete ignorance both of Robertson Smith's theories and of psycho-analysis), produced evidence 'of an ever recurring violent succession to the solitary paternal tyrant by sons, whose parricidal hands were so soon to be clenched in fratricidal strife'.[2] Freud's theory has been strongly criticized by some modern anthropologists[3] on the ground that no valid evidence exists for his totemic argument. We ought, therefore, to set out Freud's thesis in his own words:

> The Darwinian conception of the primal horde does not, of course, allow for the beginning of totemism. There is only a violent, jealous father who keeps all the females for himself and drives away the growing sons. This primal state of society has nowhere been observed. The most primitive organization we know, which to-day is still in force with certain tribes, is *associations of men* consisting of members with equal rights, subject to the restrictions of the totemic system and founded on matriarchy, or descent through the mother. Can the one have resulted from the other, and how was this possible?
>
> By basing our argument upon the celebration of the totem we are in a position to give an answer: One day the expelled brothers joined forces, slew and ate the father, and thus put an end to the horde father. Together they dared and accomplished what would have remained impossible for them singly. Perhaps some advance in culture, like the use of a new weapon, had given them the feeling of superiority. Of course these cannibalistic savages ate their victim. This violent primal father had surely been an envied and feared model for each of the brothers. The totem feast, which is perhaps mankind's first celebration, would be the repetition and commemoration of this memorable criminal act with which so many things began, social organization, moral restrictions and religion.

Freud pursued this argument as follows:

> After they [the parricides] had satisfied their hate by his removal, and had carried out their wish for identification with him, the suppressed tender impulses had to assert themselves. This took place in the form of

---

[1] See an Appendix published in Andrew Lang: *Social Origins* (1903), and A. L. Kroeber: 'Totem and Taboo – An Ethnologic Psycho-Analysis'. *American Anthropologist* Vol. XXII (1920) pp. 48–55.

[2] See Atkinson: *Primal Law* p. 220 f., quoted in Freud: *Totem and Taboo*: chap. IV.

[3] 'There is no anthropological evidence for a "dislocation in the family life of the primitive horde" as a result of the sexual urge, the sons slaying the father in order to secure the women for themselves, and then inventing a ritual device to expiate and commemorate their crime . . . at least no traces have been left of its occurrence in any known culture. . . .' E. O. James: *Comparative Religion* (1938) p. 33.

> remorse, a sense of guilt was formed which coincided here with the remorse generally felt. The dead now became stronger than the living had been, even as we observe it to-day in the destinies of men. . . . They undid their deed by declaring that the killing of the father substitute, the totem, was not allowed, and renounced the fruits of their deed by denying themselves the liberated women. Thus they created the two fundamental taboos of totemism out of the sense of guilt of the sons, and for this very reason these had to correspond with the two repressed wishes of the Oedipus Complex. Whoever disobeyed became guilty of the only two crimes which troubled primitive society.[1]

These two crimes, as Robertson Smith had suggested, are 'murder and incest, or offences of a like kind against the sacred law of blood'.[2]

But how did the feeling of guilt get handed down, by what means did this primeval crime achieve its lasting influence, so that the action of the parricides became part of the psychical structure of successive generations? Freud, in order to answer these questions, was forced to propound the theory of a mass psyche, or a collective soul.

> We base everything upon the assumption of a psyche of the mass in which psychic processes occur as in the psychic life of the individual. Moreover, we let the sense of guilt for the deed survive for thousands of years, remaining effective in generations which could not have known anything of this deed. We allow an emotional process such as might have arisen among the generations of sons that had been ill-treated by their fathers, to continue to new generations which had escaped such treatment by the very removal of the father. . . . Without the assumption of a mass psyche . . . social psychology could not exist at all. If psychic processes of one generation did not continue in the next . . . there would be no progress in this field and almost no development.[3]

In the four essays which represent a closely knit argument, Freud sets out first 'The Savage's Dread of Incest', showing the elaborate precautions which primitive tribes took in order to avoid any relationship that could be judged to be incestuous. The argument of the second essay, 'Taboo and the Ambivalence of Emotions', shows that the essence of taboo is the prohibition of contact with anything judged to be 'sacred'. Among the particular taboos discussed are those connected with leaders (kings or priests), the extraordinary ambivalence of protecting their persons and the ruthless measures taken to secure their deaths when their powers were thought to be failing. From these considerations, Freud arrived at two conclusions, first, that the emotions of primitive peoples show a greater ambivalence than do

[1] Freud: *Totem and Taboo*: Penguin edn. pp. 217–20.
[2] Robertson Smith: *Religion of the Semites* (1894) p. 419.
[3] Freud: op. cit. pp. 240–1.

those of civilized peoples, and, secondly, that the psycho-neuroses of modern patients display an inescapable likeness to the ambivalences associated with primitive taboos.

In the essay on 'Animism, Magic and the Omnipotence of Thought', Freud adopted R. R. Marett's pre-animistic stage which, Freud said, was to be identified with the practice of 'pure magic'. Marett had said that the basis of magic was a solipsist belief in the omnipotence of one's thought and wishes, a belief which Freud described as a form of primitive narcissism. But the argument reaches its climax in 'The Infantile Recurrence of Totemism' in which Freud accepted anthropological evidence that totems were originally animals, that totemism on its sexual side was related to exogamy, and that the attitude of the younger male members of primitive hordes to their horde-leaders was parricidal. Freud then proceeded to show that these anthropological occurrences have their psychological parallels in two features of the Oedipus Complex – the incestuous attraction of the mother to the son, and the death wishes directed by the son against the father.

There is another argument which Freud included in his fourth essay of great importance for our purpose, as we shall see when we come to discuss the psychology of worship, and, in particular, the psychology of 'sacrifice' as a prominent feature in man's religious activities. Sacrifice at an altar is an essential part in the ritual of all religions, and its origins appear to be the same everywhere. Originally the word 'sacrifice' referred to 'an act of social fellowship between the deity and his worshipper'. Man shared with his god the same kind of food as he himself ate, with the exception that vegetable offerings were not shared by man but left to his god. Animal sacrifices, which were undoubtedly the earliest form of sacrifice, were shared by man and deity. The members of a clan or tribe publicly participated in the rite. According to Robertson Smith

> every sacrifice was originally a clan sacrifice and the killing of a sacrificial animal originally belonged to those acts which were forbidden to the individual and were justified only if the whole kin assumed the responsibility. Primitive man had only one class of actions which were thus characterized, namely, actions which touched the holiness of the kin's common blood . . . in other words: the sacrificial animal was treated like one of kin: the sacrificing community, its god and the sacrificial animal were of the same blood, and the members of a clan.[1]

[1] Robertson Smith: quoted Freud: op. cit. p. 210.

Robertson Smith on this evidence identified the totem animal of the tribe with the sacrificial victim. The motive of this communal sacrifice is shown by Robertson Smith to be that of *participation* (always an important aspect of communal worship). 'The holy mystery of the sacrificial death was justified in that only in this way could the holy bond be established which united the participants with each other and with their god.'[1] Freud himself assumed that the totem animal was to be identified with the murdered horde-father; that totemic religion included as its two leading aspects, a sacramental killing and a communal eating of the totem sacrifice. The memory of the original murder of the horde-father defied all attempts at suppression, although the sense of guilt assumed different forms as man passed from the nomadic food-gathering stage to the settled agricultural life. Mythology makes it clear that the son who carried out the totemic sacrifice released the rest of the tribe from their sense of guilt. But, says Freud:

> There was another way of allaying this sense of guilt and this is the one that Christ took. He sacrificed his own life and thereby redeemed the brothers from primal sin. . . .
>
> In the Christian myth man's original sin is undoubtedly an offence against God the Father, and if Christ redeems mankind from the weight of original sin by sacrificing his own life, he forces us to the conclusion that this sin was murder. . . .
>
> If this sacrifice of one's own life brings about a reconciliation with god, the father, then the crime which must be expiated can only have been the murder of the father. . . . But now the psychological fatality of ambivalence demands its rights. In the same deed which offers the greatest possible expiation to the father, the son also attains the goal of his wishes against the father. He becomes a god himself beside, or rather in place of his father. The religion of the son succeeds the religion of the father. . . . Thus through the ages we see the identity of the totem feast with the animal sacrifice, the theanthropic human sacrifice, and the Christian eucharist, and in all these solemn occasions we recognize the after-effects of that crime which so oppressed men but of which they must have been so proud. At bottom, however, the Christian communion is a new setting aside of the father, a repetition of the crime that must be expiated. We see how well justified is Frazer's dictum that 'the Christian communion has absorbed within itself a sacrament which is doubtless far older than Christianity'.[2]

The significance of Freud's standpoint will become clearer when we come to discuss 'sacrifice' as an essential part of worship.

[1] Quoted Freud: op. cit. p. 212. [2] Freud: op. cit. pp. 234–7.

Criticisms

The original and contentious nature of many of Freud's theories has given rise to many incisive criticisms. One of the most searching of these criticisms deals with Freud's theory that totemism is the source of all subsequent religion. Father Wilhelm Schmidt advanced five serious objections:

1) Totemism as a practice does not belong to the earliest forms of human development. Peoples who are ethnologically the oldest have neither totemism nor totemistic sacrifice.
2) Totemism is not a universal practice. Schmidt adduced substantial evidence to show that three of the leading races of mankind, the Indo-Europeans, the Hamito-Semites, and the Ural-Altaics had originally no totemistic practices.
3) Freud's adoption of Robertson Smith's assumption that the ceremonial killing and eating of the totem animal is an essential feature of totemism is valueless. 'Of the many hundred totemic races of the whole earth there are just four who know any rite even approximating to this one and they all belong, ethnologically speaking, to the most modern totemic peoples.'
4) Pre-totemic peoples know nothing about cannibalism, so that the parricidal meal would be an impossibility.

These four objections, Schmidt summed up in a fifth objection:

5) 'The form of the pre-totemic family, and, therefore, of the earliest human family we can hope to know anything about . . . is neither general promiscuity nor group marriage, neither of which, according to the verdict of leading modern ethnologists, ever existed at all.'[1]

* * *

Another estimate of a somewhat different kind was made by Bronislaw Malinowski[2] who, as a result of his work among the Trobriand Islanders of Melanesia, his interest in psycho-analysis and his first-hand studies of matrilineal forms of society, advanced other serious criticisms of Freud's thesis. Culture and religion, said Malinowski, do not spring suddenly into being as the result of a supposed historical event but are the slow accumulation of experience. 'It is

[1] Wilhelm Schmidt: *The Origins and Growth of Religion*: Eng. trans. H. J. Rose (1935) pp. 103 ff.
[2] B. Malinowski: *Sex and Repression in Savage Society* (1937).

impossible to assume origins of culture as one creative act by which culture, fully armed, springs into being out of one crime, cataclysm or rebellion.' [1] There are also criticisms which can be offered on psychological grounds:

> If the real cause of the Oedipus complex and of culture into the bargain is to be sought in that traumatic act of birth by parricide; if the complex merely survived in the 'race memory of mankind' – then the complex ought obviously to wear out with time. On Freud's theory the Oedipus complex should have been a dreadful reality at first, a haunting memory later, but in the highest culture it should tend to disappear.[2]

In addition, Malinowski criticized Freud's patrilineal explanation of the origins of religion by comparing such systems with the matrilineal forms of the Trobriand Islanders. In the West patrilineal forms are understandably associated with the Oedipus Complex, but matrilineal societies show no feelings of hatred for the father while the infant's feelings for the mother are spontaneous and non-incestuous.

* * *

It is interesting to note, in view of what we have just quoted from Malinowski's studies of matrilineal societies, another view which was advanced by Dr Ian Suttie.[3] Discussing the Painted Pottery cultures which once extended from North China to Spain (cultures whose social life was organized around a temple in each village), Suttie says that their myth-and-ritual pattern expresses the same child attitude as modern analytical studies show to be operative in individual lives today, although this child-attitude no longer exercises a dominant influence in society. The deity was not a Sky-Father but an Earth-Mother, indicating that the worshippers were mother-directed rather than father-directed. Crimes, therefore, were offences against the mother and not, as in Freud's primal hordes, against the sexual privileges of the horde-father. The 'theology' of the Earth-Mother expressed a pre-Oedipal attitude to the Mother who was regarded as being both good and terrible, and, therefore, aroused ambivalent emotions. The sacrificial theme of matrilineal religion was different from that of patrilineal cults, the 'god' being treated with high honours before being offered as the sacrificial 'child' victim to the Earth-Mother. The sexual element was, therefore, not so pro-

[1] Malinowski: op. cit. p. 167. [2] op. cit. pp. 167–8.
[3] Ian Suttie: *The Origins of Love and Hate* (1939).

minent as in patrilineal totem sacrifices, since the Earth-Mother was the source both of children and of food.

When in the cultural history of the race the fathers supplanted the mothers, the Sky-Father supplanted the Earth-Mother and the victim of the sacrificial ritual who had died to support the life of the people, became a scapegoat for the sins of parricidal and incestuously inclined males. From this Suttie proceeded to show that religion instead of being an obsessional neurosis of guilt was a form of psycho-social therapy – that human life instead of being dominated by hate was regenerated and united by love.

* * *

Moses and Monotheism

Freud's last psychological explanation of religion is contained in the book he completed in London as a highly respected refugee from the Nazi invasion of Austria, *Moses and Monotheism* (1939). This book covers a much wider range of interests than its title at first suggests, for it is concerned not only with Jewish religion but with Christianity and religion in general. It will be well to begin with a brief account of Freud's use of Old Testament references to Moses, before pursuing Freud's psychological argument. Freud suggested that since Moses is an Egyptian name[1] the Moses of the Exodus was an Egyptian not a Hebrew. But if so, then why was the child delivered to the waters of the Nile? There are many myths which deal with the practice of child-exposure, so that this Biblical incident would seem to belong to this mythical pattern, but this does not help us to decide whether the child was Egyptian or Hebrew. It is said that he was brought up as the son of an Egyptian princess. If so, we have to ask why should Moses, brought up in an Egyptian palace, have joined the enslaved Hebrew community? The answer, according to Freud, is that by adopting the Hebrews as his own people, and by imposing upon them the knowledge of the One True God and leading them out of Egypt, Moses was able to secure the survival of the new religion which had been introduced by Amenhotep IV who is better known as Ikhnaton. The introduction of monotheism into Egypt was violently repudiated by the Egyptian priesthood after Ikhnaton's death but survived, outside Egypt, as the result of Moses' efforts with the Hebrews after the

[1] The Egyptian word is Mose(s) – the final 's' being a Greek addition. The Hebrew form is Mosheh.

Exodus. During the period in the wilderness Moses was subject to various rebellious uprisings against his authority and in the end Moses was murdered.[1] The memory of that murder was, according to Freud, suppressed for many centuries; the revival of this memory was to prove of great importance for Christianity.

We need not consider at any length the objections which Biblical scholars have directed against this thesis. There is no reliable evidence to support the view that Moses was associated with Ikhnaton's reign nor his religious reformation.[2] Further the statement that evidence for the murder of Moses is to be found in the book of the prophet Hosea has been denied by most scholars. The importance of Sellin's statement lies in the use which Freud made of this supposed fact, namely that the revived knowledge of the 'murder' of Moses and, many centuries later, the crucifixion of Jesus, released the suppressed memories of the ancestral murder of the horde-leader.

> I invite the reader to take a step forward and assume that in the history of the human species something happened similar to the events in the life of the individual. That is to say, mankind as a whole passed through conflicts of a sexual-aggressive nature, which left permanent traces but which were for the most part warded off and forgotten; later, after a long period of latency, they came to life again and created phenomena similar in structure and tendency to neurotic symptoms.[3]

All religions are characterized by fixations 'on the old family history' and 'by reproductions of the past and a return long after of what had been forgotten'.[4] Behind the historical developments of Judaism lie the repressed memories of the murder of the primal father, memories which were brought back into consciousness by such 'events' as the murder of Moses. The result was a strong revival of feelings of guilt among the Jewish people, feelings which reached their fullest expression in the doctrines of Paul of Tarsus who traced this widespread feeling of guilt, as he experienced it under the catharsis of the death of Jesus of Nazareth, to its primeval source. The Christ-figure assumed the long remembered, long forgotten, guilt of the brothers

[1] Freud here adopted a doubtful opinion put forward by E. Sellin: *Mose und seine Bedeutung fuer die israelitisch-juedische Religionsgeschichte* (1922).

[2] One of the most serious difficulties arises from the dating of the Exodus and the reign of Ikhnaton. Dr H. L. Philp: *Freud and Religious Belief* (1956) has set out these chronological difficulties fully, see pp. 103–15. None of the dates given for the Exodus by well-known Old Testament scholars would support the idea that Moses was a disciple of Ikhnaton or a personal supporter of his monotheism.

[3] Freud: *Moses and Monotheism* (1939) p. 129.

[4] op. cit. p. 136.

who were responsible for the murder of the horde-father. This is a point we have already noted in Freud's *Totem and Taboo*.

Consequences

Although Freud's conclusions aroused much opposition, it is noteworthy that the arguments have not discouraged many writers from employing Freudian concepts both in their studies of religion and in pastoral activities. Canon L. W. Grensted points out that C. H. Valentine in his *Modern Psychology and the Validity of Christian Experience* (1926), and he himself in his Bampton Lectures (1930) on *Psychology and God*, were among the earliest of English writers who 'saw that the importance of Freud's methods and their validity in applied psycho-analysis did not necessitate the conclusions which he drew from them, but might well be interpreted in quite a different way'.[1] Freud's views that religion is a neurosis did not antagonize Oskar Pfister of Zurich, a Protestant pastor-theologian well known to English readers.[2] Pfister was not so much interested in Freud's psychological explanations about the nature of religion as in the Freudian technique of relieving those psychological disorders which impaired the religious life. Pfister's main thesis is that the deviations of Christianity as an historical movement are attributable to psychical errors:

> When it is measured against the principle laid down by Jesus in the Gospel according to Saint John . . . the history of Christianity rather has the appearance of a gigantic misunderstanding or of a pathology of Christianity. In its frequently savage attachment to an irrational dogma having no connection with love, dogmatics and its history seemed to me to constitute an attempt to evade the central point of Jesus's teaching and claims. I saw men terrified by the letter of the Gospel and the tenets of the Church, any questioning of which was threatened by the stake and hell fire. . . .[3]

He goes on to give an account of how he looked for some means of curing these defects of Christianity in the lives of people known to him, and found himself powerfully attracted by Freud's psycho-analytic view that neuroses are caused by conflicts of conscience repressed within the unconscious which, unless treated successfully by psycho-analytic methods, powerfully affect men's lives for ill.

[1] L. W. Grensted: *The Psychology of Religion* (1952) p. 58.

[2] See Oskar Pfister: *Some Applications of Psycho-Analysis* (1923) and *Christianity and Fear* (1948).

[3] Pfister: op. cit. p. 22.

While unable to accept Freud's atheistic and materialistic views, Pfister was greatly attracted by their psychological value. 'The study of fear and compulsion neuroses and of their effect on religion and ethical life opened my eyes to important complexes of fact and the laws governing them. . . . The neurosis of individuals leads to a neurotic malformation of their Christian faith. . . .'[1] Pfister's analyses, as a working pastor, were more or less confined to treating adolescents troubled by moral conflicts, and he was able to supplement his procedures by moral and religious advice. In a letter which Freud wrote to Pfister, for whom he had a lively appreciation, there are two sentences which help us to understand how it was that Pfister, and others like him, have found the Freudian techniques so helpful without sharing Freud's views about the nature of religion. Freud writes:

> In itself psycho-analysis is neither religious nor the opposite, but an impartial instrument which can serve the clergy as well as the laity when it is used only to free suffering people. I have been very struck at realizing how I had never thought of the extraordinary help the psycho-analytic method can be in pastoral work, probably because wicked heretics like us are so far away from that circle.[2]

We are, therefore, confronted with a paradoxical situation. As a technique psycho-analysis has proved itself to be of great value in pastoral work – more so among Protestants than among Catholics, and that for reasons we shall discuss later[3] – but as an explanation applied to religion its real contribution lies not so much in what it denies as in the lively and positive interpretations which such views have provoked,[4] particularly among theologians. It is, therefore, a matter of some regret that Jung among others should have underestimated the value of these responses to the Freudian views by saying how surprised he was that so many clergy should have sought practical help from Freud's theory of sexuality: 'these theories are hostile to spiritual values . . . they are rational methods of treatment which actually hinder the realization of meaningful experience'.[5]

[1] op. cit. pp. 23–4.
[2] See Ernest Jones: *Sigmund Freud*: Vol. III. p. 312, and also letter dated 9th Feb. 1909 quoted by Jones: op. cit. Vol. II. pp. 489–90.
[3] See pp. 97 ff.
[4] Ernest Jones gives a brief but interesting résumé of the reactions of certain Anglican writers to Freud's analytical views on religion, quoting with particular approval those by Dr R. S. Lee in his *Freud and Christianity* (1948). Jones: op. cit. Vol. III. pp. 386–8.
[5] Jung: *Modern Man in Search of a Soul* (1936) p. 263.

Some General Conclusions

We have seen how difficult it is to define religion, but Freud's 'natural atheism' caused him to define its nature much too narrowly. It is true that man is vividly aware, even under the protective screens of civilization, of a general and individual insecurity, but this does not justify our describing man's attitude to the universe as being consequently neurotic. Erich Fromm may believe that religion has its origin 'in man's helplessness in confronting the forces of nature outside and the instinctive forces within himself',[1] and that this anxiety often characterizes those suffering from some form of neurosis. He may urge, as Freud did, that 'Man must educate himself to face reality and to do so he must overcome the infantile fixation of still being a child in his father's house. We must grow up and think for ourselves.' [2] But this feeling of insecurity is not necessarily an adult regression to the fears of childhood. It could be argued that this feeling is a sign of man's recognition of a *separation* between himself, other selves, and God.

> Man's greatest happiness is experienced in those moments when his perception of himself as a separate individuality is at its lowest. . . . All happiness is a little death, in which the individual abandons for the moments of its duration the conglomeration of desires, sentiments and ambitions which go to make up his personality.[3]

Man feels himself to be safe when he recovers a sense of religious conviction founded not only on custom and inherited traditions, but also on experience and revelation. It is the limitation of the Freudian approach to religion that it has no place for religious experience and none for supernatural revelation; that in its emphasis upon the determinism of the father-son relationship it overlooks the need which man has had at every level of culture for explanations and interpretations of life itself. Man has a deep craving for some kind of metaphysical belief. Freud had it himself, otherwise he would not have been so preoccupied with the psychology of an activity in which he did not believe. This craving is an adult need not a regression to an infantile attitude. It is well to remember that 'we need not assert either the absolute reality of religious content or that religion is a flight from intolerable reality. . . . Religion is not one thing, but many, and we as psychologists are in no position to make easy assertions about its manifest contents.' [4]

[1] Erich Fromm: *Psycho-Analysis and Religion* (1951) pp. 18–19.
[2] op. cit. p. 21. [3] Arthur Guirdham: *Christ and Freud* (1959) pp. 15–16.
[4] Michael Fordham: *The Objective Psyche* (1958) p. 41.

Chapter VII

JUNG ON RELIGION

Jung, unlike Freud who maintained a clear-cut, critical attitude towards religion, despite his sympathetic approach, has so frequently reassessed his attitudes as to make it difficult to give a really consistent account of his position.[1] Jung always refused to consider his voluminous output as a 'system'. 'I regard my theories as suggestions and attempts at the formulation of a new scientific concept of psychology, based in the first place upon immediate experience with human beings.' [2] Yet in spite of this, the value of Jung's contribution exceeds that of any other writer on this subject in this century. We have already considered some of the more important of Jung's psychological concepts[3] so that we are now free to make, first, a brief résumé of Jung's personal record, an assessment of the significance of his views on theology and religion and then a comparison (based partly on his own estimate)[4] between his attitude to religion and that of Freud.

Personal Record

Carl Gustav Jung was born in Kesswil, Switzerland, in 1875. His father was a Protestant pastor and a philologist. Jung wished at first to become an archaeologist (a wish that may be interpreted symbolically as a desire to delve into the unexplored places of human experience), but later he took a medical degree at Basel intending to specialize in physiological chemistry. A chance reading of Krafft-Ebing's *Text*

[1] Professor Raymond Hostie stresses the fact that 'Jung himself [has] never published any general bird's eye view of his psychological ideas to which reference can be made'. Raymond Hostie: *Religion and the Psychology of Jung* (1957) p. 4.
Professor Hostie's book contains a particularly useful bibliography of Jung's works with the dates of their publication in German and the corresponding dates and titles of English translations or rearrangements of separate articles and essays.

[2] Jung's foreword to Jolande Jacobi: *The Psychology of C. G. Jung* (1942).

[3] See chaps. IV and V.

[4] See Jung: *Freud and Psycho-analysis*: Collected Works: Vol. 4 (1961).

Book of Psychiatry led him to become an assistant at the Burghölzli Asylum in Zurich, where he collaborated with Eugen Bleuler, later going to Paris for a short time to study under Janet. His use in Zurich of a new method known as Association Tests helped him to confirm empirically some of Freud's published conclusions so that from 1907 there was a fruitful collaboration between them which later led to disagreement, and ended with the publication of Jung's *Psychology of the Unconscious* (1912). From this time onwards Jung ceased to be associated with the Freudian psycho-analytical school, establishing his own approach under the title of Analytical Psychology.[1]

In the years that followed Jung found that his knowledge of the nature of the unconscious was increased by visits to primitive tribes in North Africa, Arizona, New Mexico and Kenya. As a result of these ethnological researches, Jung found striking similarities between the myth-and-ritual patterns of primitive peoples, the religions of classical antiquity and the contents of the unconscious of his patients. This interest in non-European tribal customs and religions was later extended to include the great religions of the East which resulted in his association with Richard Wilhelm in *The Secret of the Golden Flower* (1931) and with C. Kerényi in *Essays on Science of Mythology* (1941). Jung from his boyhood had been deeply impressed with the mystery of existence, and he tells how quite early in life he became interested in the subtleties of theology.

> I well remember my confirmation lessons at the hands of my father. The catechism bored me unspeakably. Once I turned the leaves of the little book in order to find something of interest and my glance fell on the paragraphs about the Trinity. That interested me, and I waited impatiently till the instruction had advanced to that section. But when the longed-for lesson had arrived, my father said, 'We will skip this section; I cannot make anything out of it myself.' With that my last hope was laid in the grave.[2]

Jung's interest in this particular aspect of theology none the less survived this youthful disappointment; many years later he published his 'Psychological Approach to the Dogma of the Trinity'.[3] Another

[1] The history of this collaboration reveals misunderstandings on both sides. Two quite different accounts of these 'dissensions' are given by Ernest Jones: *Sigmund Freud*: Vol. II (1955) pp. 155 ff., and by E. A. Bennet: *C. G. Jung* (1961) pp. 33 ff.

[2] Jung: *Integration of the Personality* (1940) p. 64.

[3] See *Psychology and Religion: West and East*: Collected Works: Vol. 11. pp. 107 ff.

youthful experience which, Jung says, profoundly affected his adult attitude to religion was a dream which he had at about the age of twelve. He dreamed that he was standing in the gloomy medieval courtyard of the Gymnasium at Basel and as he went out through the great gateway he saw

> the Cathedral of Basel, the sun shining on the roof of coloured tiles, recently renovated, a most impressive sight. Above the Cathedral, God was sitting on His throne. I thought: 'How beautiful it all is! What a wonderful world this is – how perfect, how complete, how full of harmony.' Then something happened, so unexpectedly and so shattering that I woke up. There the dream ended. I could not allow myself to *think* of what I had seen.

For the next few nights he felt it would be an 'unforgivable sin' to think the thought he had had in that dream.

> Then came a great moment: he sat up in bed, sweating and trembling, for he felt: 'God must mean me to accept this awful scene as my own thought,' and at that moment he did accept it. It was as follows: From His throne God 'dropped' a vast faeces on the Cathedral and smashed it to pieces. This was a terrific thing, for it could only mean that the Church, his father's teaching, and his own beliefs had to be thought of in an entirely different way, because God had poured scorn on every one of them.[1]

Dr Bennet, commenting upon this experience, says that this was a 'great' dream in that it seems to have convinced Jung that he must take an independent attitude to religion, a conviction which subsequently dominated the whole of his outlook, as his life's work manifestly proves.

During his association with Freud, Jung produced a small work, 'The Significance of the Father in the Destiny of the Individual' (1909),[2] in which he expressed views agreeing with those of Freud:

> What we see in the development of the world-process, the original sources of the changes in the Godhead, we see also in the individual. Parental power guides the child like a higher controlling fate. But when he begins to grow up, there begins also the conflict between the infantile constellation and the individual; the parental influence dating from the prehistoric (infantile) period is repressed, sinks into the unconscious but is not thereby eliminated . . . Like everything that has passed into the unconscious, the infantile constellation sends up into consciousness, dim, foreboding feelings, feelings of mysterious guidance and opposing

---

[1] E. A. Bennet: *C. G. Jung* (1961) pp. 16 ff.

[2] See Jung: *Freud and Psycho-analysis*: Collected Works: Vol. 4. pp. 301 ff.

> influences. Here are the roots of the first religious sublimations. In the place of the father, with his constellating virtues and faults, there appears on the one hand, an altogether sublime deity, on the other the devil. . . .[1]

But Jung's views were soon to undergo a considerable change. His attempts to deal with the phenomena of religion as objective psychical 'facts' led him to the conclusion that the psychological processes at work in modern believers were the same as those which operated in pre-Christian and non-Christian religions. All religions have their psychological roots in the collective unconscious of the race.

Jung and Theology

Jung's views, despite their positive nature, have aroused profound doubts among many theologians as to whether he might not be identifying psychical facts with spiritual realities. It is difficult, for instance, to reconcile such a statement as the following with the teaching of traditional theology:

> To our analytical psychology . . . the image of God is the symbolic expression of a certain psychological state, or function, which has the character of absolute superiority to the conscious will of the subject. . . . God is a function of the unconscious, namely the manifestation of a split-off sum of libido which has activated the God-imago. To the orthodox view God is, of course, absolute, i.e., existing in Himself. Such a conception implies a complete severance from the unconscious, which means, psychologically, a complete unawareness of the fact that the divine effect springs from one's inner self.[2]

Again, theologians find it difficult to accept the view that

> It is only through the psyche that we can establish that God acts upon us, but we are unable to distinguish whether these actions emanate from God or from the unconscious. We cannot tell whether God and the unconscious are two different entities. Both are border-line concepts for transcendental contents.[3]

particularly when Jung declares that by 'God' he means the 'God-image' (God-*imago*) and that by 'transcendental' he implies a transition from one attitude to another and not any metaphysical quality.[4] These difficulties arose in the first place from certain ambiguities in the *Psychology of the Unconscious*. Although Jung assumed that religion is psychologically irreplaceable he implied that once a man had succeeded in becoming psychologically integrated he became

[1] op. cit. [2] Jung: *Psychological Types* (1938) pp. 300–1.
[3] Jung: *Answer to Job* (1954) p. 177: and Collected Works: Vol. 11. pp. 468–9.
[4] See Jung: *Psychological Types* (1923) p. 610.

spiritually autonomous. On the other hand, Jung's use of the term 'undifferentiated libido', as distinct from the Freudian sexual libido, necessitated a more favourable orientation of theological opinion about the nature of analytical theories.[1]

Jung on many occasions protested that his theological critics overlooked the fact that his *methodology* – his gathering of observable facts and his elaboration of their psychical nature – was of the same empirical nature as the methods of modern science. To this empirical approach, Jung in the course of time added the factor of faith. This addition was the result of his conviction – a conviction based on analytical practice – that the psychical phenomena of his patients, and the information which his ethnological researches had brought to him, showed that all men live for some end whether they are conscious of it or not. Life is a *drama* in which plot, word, action and gesture are to be interpreted *prospectively.* The end to which the drama moves is what Jung calls the Self. (We have already referred to this in our note on Individuation.) But there is a paradox here. The Self, which is the goal of the individual life, is also the goal of all other individual lives even as Christ may be said to be the goal of one man's life and at the same time the goal of all men's lives. From the theological standpoint, misunderstanding of Jung's *prospective* interpretation arises from the fact that Jung applied to the Self the same adjectives as Otto applied to the *numinosum* – *mysterium,* in the sense of that which is wholly Other (*das ganz Andere*), *tremendum,* in the sense of that which is possessed of a powerful and sometimes destructive nature, and *fascinans,* in the sense of a Goal to which men feel themselves to be drawn. Such a Self appears to be a substitute for God, although it should be borne in mind that many of the greatest mystics often referred to the Self in terms of the God resident in man. For many mystics, as for St Paul, this Self is the Christ-who-lives-in-me, but when we are referring to human experience it must be remembered that the Self cannot be that totality which is God.[2]

Another possible objection, theologically, arises from Jung's inter-

[1] Father Victor White points out that this 'undifferentiated libido' could be synonymous with that formless energy which natural theology knows as *actus purus,* which is a conception of God Himself. Jung's prospectively directed libido could be interpreted as that *naturale desiderium* which St Thomas Aquinas assumed men have to reach out towards God. See Victor White: *God and the Unconscious* (1952) p. 50.

[2] In answer to the objection that this conception of the Self seems to provide a psychological substitute for God, Jung protests: 'I have never anywhere denied

est in the nature of the Trinity and his proposal that such a Trinity must be psychologically a Quaternity (*Tetraktys*). The nature of the fourth member is not wholly clear; it may be the Shadow, or the darkness that is opposed to the light, or moral evil (*malum*) as opposed to goodness. But if the fourth member of the Quaternity is identified with evil, then the Godhead embodies the principle of evil. Such a belief is opposed to the traditional view – *malum est privatio boni.* Professor Raymond Hostie, discussing this view, says that

> The evil that Jung is concerned with is . . . pre-eminently psychic. But we must understand what this word means. Psychic evil includes external events independent of the person suffering them, as well as the purely objective inner realities that are hampering his development. [But] Jung often calls psychic evil a moral evil. In doing so, he gives this latter phrase a meaning not sanctioned by the traditional terminology, which uses it to mean sin. For Jung moral evil is evil that attacks the psyche. . . .

But Jung attacked the theory of evil as *privatio boni,*

> as something that destroyed the reality of evil wherever he met it – in Greek philosophy, and in the Church Fathers, particularly St Augustine whom he accuses of taking it from the Greeks to get round his own Manicheism. Jung by postulating that good and evil are found together in God, believes he escapes from the dualism that seems inevitable when one stresses the real, positive, character of evil as strongly as he does.[1]

Evil in Christian theology is closely allied with the existence of matter, and matter, as Jung points out, is psychologically associated with the feminine principle. This masculine-feminine association of Good-and-Evil has its parallel in Hindu metaphysics where Brahman manifested as Siva (the heavenly principle often represented by the phallic symbol) is also manifested as Sakto, the female earthly principle. This leads Jung to say that the fourth principle is the Mother who with the (masculine) Trinity completes the Figure of Quaternity.[2]

God. I proceed from a positive Christianity, which is as much Catholic as it is Protestant, and I endeavour to demonstrate, in a scientific and responsible manner, those facts which can be ascertained empirically and which not only lend plausibility to the Christian dogma, and especially the Catholic dogma, but are also likely to provide scientifically-minded people with some way towards understanding it. . . .' Footnote from a letter dated 22 September 1944: quoted by Professor Gebhard Frei in Victor White: *God and the Unconscious* (1952) p. 258.

[1] Raymond Hostie: *Religion and the Psychology of Jung* (1957) pp. 189 ff.

[2] See Jung: *Answer to Job* (1954) pp. 165–78; and Collected Works: Vol. 11. pp. 461–9. See also H. L. Philp: *Jung and the Problem of Evil* (1958) Part I: pp. 31–84, where this problem is discussed in great detail.

If the Mother is assumed into the Heavens as Queen, then, says Jung, matter itself is spiritualized in a cosmic integration of matter and spirit, which has its counterpart in the integration of the human psyche.[1]

Jung and Religion

In one of the best assessments of Jung's psychology of religion, Dr Hans Schaer quotes Professor Adolf Keller, a well-known Protestant theologian, as saying:

> The problem of religion has gradually acquired a ubiquity in Jung's thought that has no need of words to make itself felt. Where there is a soul there is also religion – not, however, in the sense of an accepted ecclesiastical form, but of a fate-like encounter with a stronger spiritual reality which compels examination. If religion as generally understood rests on one's capacity to let oneself be profoundly affected by powers that transcend consciousness, then the first and essential thing about it is this influence and not the intellectual formulation of such experiences; for the formulation is bound to be made *a posteriori* on a plane that is alien to them. The reality of these seizures is prior to the truth of their conscious formulation. Jung has once more made room for this reality in psychology.[2]

Religion for Jung, as we have seen, is not a matter confined to creedal acceptances:

> By the term 'religion' I do not mean a creed. It is, however, true that on the one hand every confession is originally based upon the experience of the numinosum and on the other upon *pistis*, the loyalty, trust and confidence towards a definitely experienced numinous effect and the subsequent alteration of consciousness: the conversion of Paul is a striking example of this. 'Religion', it might be said, is the term that designates the attitude peculiar to a consciousness which has been altered by the experience of the numinosum.[3]

---

[1] Jung supported this view in his extended study of Alchemy: see *Psychology and Alchemy*: Collected Works. Vol. 12, which has as a frontispiece a picture of 'The Creator as Ruler of the Threefold and the Fourfold Universe, with fire and water as the counterpart of heaven'. From the *Theatrum Chemicum Britannicum* 9. p. 210.

Another illustration of this Quaternity appears as the frontispiece of Collected Works: Vol. 11, from *The Book of Hours of Etienne Chevalier* (Chantilly), showing three identical male figures as the Trinity and a female figure surrounded by an adoring host.

[2] Adolf Keller: *Die kulturelle Bedeutung der komplexen Psychologie* (1935), quoted in Hans Schaer: *Religion and the Cure of Souls in Jung's Psychology* (1951) pp. 7–8.

[3] Jung: *Psychology and Religion: West and East*: Collected Works: Vol. 11. p. 7.

Religion is, therefore, a matter of experience; man knows God not as a theological concept but as an experience from which concepts may subsequently be formulated. It is for this reason that Jung refers to God as the God-imago or God-symbol since a symbol by its very nature is able to reveal 'reality' in a way no other medium can. This does not mean that 'God' is nothing-but a psychic event within the unconscious; Jung has more than once been careful to point out that *what exists in the psyche exists in reality.*[1] Here again Jung's views appear to be in direct opposition to traditional beliefs. God, for Christian belief, is 'absolute', but if God is absolute then He cannot be that God for whom men yearn. Jung's position is that God to be 'psychologically real' cannot be 'absolute' because the Absolute cannot be known experientially, and he supports this contention by referring to a saying of Meister Eckhart (1260–1327) who believed that God is born in the soul continuously. 'God's being is of the soul, but his Godhead is of Himself.' In other words, this German mystic believed that God is 'a working function of the soul' and the soul itself a working function of the Godhead.[2] The God that is in the soul (God-imago) is that reality which we meet in religious experience, while the Godhead is that which is beyond our experience and beyond all human comprehension. On this matter psychology can say nothing.

Jung on Catholic and Protestant Christianity

It does not seem to be generally realized that the divisions of Christendom have psychological as well as theological and historical explanations. As a movement, the Reformation was not so much an attempt to modify or reform Catholic belief and practice, as the presentation of a new psychological outlook on man and religion. Psychologically the Reformation began with such radical reassessments of historical Christianity as were implied by Meister Eckhart's declaration that man can know God only as an experience in his own soul. Hitherto, for most men, the Church had been a psychological

[1] 'When I say, as a psychologist, that God is an archetype, I mean by that the *type* in the psyche. The word "type" is, as we know, derived from τύπος, "blow" or "imprint": thus an archetype presupposes a printer. . . . The religious point of view puts the accent on the imprinter, whereas scientific psychology emphasises the *typos*, the imprint, the only thing it can understand.' See Jung: *Psychology and Alchemy*: Collected Works: Vol. 12. pp. 12–17.

[2] This matter is discussed at great length in *Answer to Job* (1954), see Collected Works: Vol. 11. pp. 456 ff. and 483 ff.: also *Two Essays on Analytical Psychology*: Collected Works: Vol. 7. pp. 233–7.

necessity since, as an institution, it was a massive constellation of those symbols by which man was able to experience communally (at a remove) that reality which, if encountered directly and individually, might otherwise overwhelm him. In other words, the Church was not only the greatest objectification of religious symbolism in the history of the West, it was also the means whereby man in his religious life could be protected against archetypal invasions from the collective unconscious. Two conclusions follow from this psychological estimate of the Church. Symbols are the most vitally effective means of spiritual communication and experience; and, secondly, the Church itself as a spiritual community is the means whereby the individual enjoys a 'safe' and properly authenticated experience of reality. Both of these beliefs were rejected at the Protestant Reformation.

The social and intellectual changes of the fifteenth and sixteenth centuries had made the hitherto long-accepted symbolism of the Church irrelevant for large masses of people. This change of what is known as *symbolic attitude* reduced Catholic symbolism to a meaningless confusion of images. When a symbol loses its meaning it may continue as an historical *sign* but as a symbol it is dead. It was this rejection of 'dead' symbols that caused Jung to describe the Reformation as a form of *psychological iconoclasm*. It might equally well be described as an unusually energetic 'spring-cleaning' of symbolical rejects. The men who destroyed images and altar-pieces, and hurled stones through medieval stained-glass windows, were not merely aesthetic vandals, but men who were violently ejecting the external expressions of a symbolism which for them had died internally. Symbols are effective only so long as they are relevant to life.

This psychological iconoclasm has its connexion with the first fully Protestant affirmation – Meister Eckhart's assertion that 'God's being is in the soul'. If God (or, to use the Jungian term, the God-imago) is a function of the soul, then individual experience and not an historical Institution is the primary factor in religion. When a man believes that he can have *in his own soul* a personal experience of God, he may no longer feel the need for an organized spiritual institution – the Church. And if the Church is no longer felt to be an essential factor in his life then any sanction which the individual may subsequently need to support his experiences will have to be sought for elsewhere. Protestantism found such alternative sanctions in the Bible. But, as Jung points out, the Bible has never (partly because of the difficulties of reconciling various scholastic interpretations) had for post-Reformation churches the same authority as that of the pre-Reformation Church. It is this absence of an all-comprehensive authority which has been in large measure responsible for the continuing divisions in Christendom. But this disintegration has had a double effect. First, and negatively, 'If it [Protestantism] goes on disintegrating as a Church, it must have the effect of stripping man of all his spiritual safeguards and means of defence against immediate experience of the forces waiting for liberation in the unconscious.' [1] According to Jung, many of the neuroses which attack people in the post-Reformation world of the West arise from the fact that they are unable to establish the kind of relationship with their unconscious that would permit them to live without fear. Fear arises whenever the individual is unable to cope with some essential activity of the unconscious. When the conscious mind has repudiated symbols which in the past have been the means of 'reducing' pressures from the unconscious, the individual is subject to fear and danger. But if the Protestant has to face life without some form of insulation against invasions from the collective unconscious, he is laid open to the possibility of some unique experience of the divine.

Protestantism on its positive side is a great spiritual adventure.

> The Protestant is left to God alone. . . . If a Protestant survives the complete loss of his Church and still remains a Protestant, that is, a person who is defenceless against God and no longer protected by walls or communities – then he has a unique spiritual opportunity for immediate religious experience.[2]

Should this opportunity be fulfilled the individual becomes spiritually autonomous, a religiously integrated personality, a 'new' man, a converted personality, all that Jung implies by the term Individuation.

* * *

An Interim Judgement

Jung's views on the nature of the psychical forces involved in dogma, myth-and-ritual and experience gain an additional value from the fact that they have stimulated many religious people to view their traditional attitudes in the light of contemporary psychology. Many a man, says Jung, has need of something which personal religious

[1] Jung: *Psychology and Religion*: Collected Works: Vol. 11. p. 48.
[2] op. cit. pp. 49–50.

experience could provide but which his acquaintance with organized forms of traditional religion has not so far provided. If God is a psychical fact then man, in his experience of the God-imago in his own soul, can be aware of a *raison d'être* of which he was formerly unaware. No man can be psychologically an integrated personality, or a spiritually happy soul, unless he has some purpose to live for, some object to be united with. But – and this is the source of many conflicting views about the significance of Jung's estimate of religion – how these psychological facts are to be related to 'objective' truth is a question that remains unanswered. Jung at no time professed to be a metaphysician, although metaphysics were never far removed from his mind. 'Religion, in particular, theology, looks at the phenomena from its metaphysical position and comes to conclusions about the nature of God: psychology looks at them from the theory of the collective unconscious and comes to conclusions about human nature.' [1] Yet it is a basic belief in many religions that the nature of God and the nature of man are not two but one. A view which some of Jung's arguments would seem to support.

Freud and Jung on Religion – a Contrast

In the *Kölnische Zeitung* for 7 May 1929, there appeared an article by Jung which he later remodelled and which will be found in one of the best known of all Jung's works in English – *Modern Man in Search of a Soul.*[2] Jung opened his article by saying that 'The difference between Freud's views and my own ought really to be dealt with by someone who stands outside the circle of influence of those ideas which go under our respective names.' [3] Indeed this has been attempted by many writers, but it may be doubted whether any interested person could claim 'to be outside the circles of influence' of either Freud or Jung. Jung reminds us that some people see things differently from other people because of their own particular psychological constitution. Freud, according to Jung, interpreted the nature of man too exclusively in terms of his defects; Freud was unable to understand the real nature of religion because he interpreted everything in terms of the neurotic mind. Freud overlooked the fact that all men have need of some external check on their conclusions, even

[1] Michael Fordham: *The Objective Psyche* (1958) p. 115.

[2] Also included in Collected Works: *Freud and Psycho-Analysis*: Vol. 4. pp. 333 ff.

[3] Jung: op. cit. Collected Works: Vol. 4. p. 333.

if these conclusions be drawn from empirical data, because the individual research worker is influenced both by his own temperament and the limitations of experience and outlook. 'Knowledge rests not upon truth alone, but upon error also.' [1] This does not mean that the differences between Freud and Jung are to be regarded purely as a matter of temperament or difference of personal background; many of the differences are of a strictly logical nature. Freud believed that psychology would eventually succeed in explaining religion away in much the same way as a neurosis can be dispelled and the patient cured. Man, for Freud, needs to be cured of the neurosis of religion. Jung, on the other hand, seems to have realized quite early in life that religion is an essential activity of man and that psychology instead of seeking to explain religion away must attempt to explain how man's nature reacts to situations normally described as religious.

Another essential difference arises in connexion with the nature of the instincts. Freud said that instincts are chiefly sexual in nature (though, as we have already observed, sexuality for Freud had a larger connotation than it has for some of his critics). Jung interpreted instincts in a more general way as the source of psychical energy, saying that human behaviour is the result of a collusion between psychical energy and spirit, adding that we are as far from knowing what instinct is as we are from knowing the real nature of spirit. Because of his use of such words as 'spirit' and 'faith' Jung has been accused by some Freudian critics of being 'mystical' rather than scientific in his outlook. But Jung protests that it would be 'unscientific' to overlook the fact that the mystical idea 'is enforced by the natural tendencies of the unconscious mind'.[2] In turn, he himself criticized Freud's concept of the Super-Ego, saying that it was nothing more than a furtive attempt 'to smuggle in his time-honoured image of Jehovah in the dress of a psychological theory'.[3] For Jung libidinal energy is that which moves prospectively to a new birth, to some reorientation of purpose, and not as with Freud, regressively or incestuously as in the Oedipus Complex.

Behind all individual expressions of libidinal activity there are, says Jung, the phylogenetic contents of the collective unconscious; it is the archetypal figure of the Father-God operating within the unconscious that causes the child to regard the human father as the

[1] op. cit. p. 336.
[2] See *Psychology and Religion*: Collected Works: Vol. 11. p. 58.
[3] *Freud and Psycho-analysis*: Collected Works: Vol. 4. p. 339.

God-image and not the other way round, as Freud had contended. Man, for Jung, outgrows the infantile stage of religion by becoming aware that his life and thought are affected by archetypal activities which bring the contents of experience within a religious purview. Instead of regarding phantasies and symbols as means whereby the individual seeks to avoid 'reality' (which was Freud's view) Jung accepted such phenomena as 'symbols of transformation'.[1] In other words, all such symbols are for Jung the means by which man gains a knowledge (*gnosis*) of realities which are *in themselves* unknowable – realities which cannot be comprehended in any other way.

For Freud religion was an obsessional neurosis, and at no time did he modify that judgement. For Jung it was the absence of religion that was the chief cause of adult psychological disorders. These two sentences indicate how great is the difference between their respective standpoints on religion.

[1] This is the title under which *The Psychology of the Unconscious* now appears in Jung's Collected Works, Vol. 5.

Part II

PSYCHOLOGY AND RELIGIOUS PRACTICES

Chapter VIII

THE GROWTH OF RELIGIOUS CONSCIOUSNESS

In the section on 'Original Monotheism' we noted a suggestion that primitive man formed a notion of the Infinite from his experience of things of which his senses could perceive no limit, and that this experiential sense of the Infinite had its parallel in the religious development of young children who associated Big Beings with Big Things.

The Child and God

If we compare the development of the very young child with that of primitive peoples we see that there is a level of consciousness at which both have a sense of lurking mystery which is later known as 'God'.

> At what age does the child begin to make for himself a concept of God? That is a problem which does not lend itself to precise and absolute solution. We may say, however, that in the generality of cases the first manifestations of the religious idea present themselves at the age of questioning, that is to say towards the age of three.[1]

This intellectualization of his growing sense of curiosity and wonder, and his developing religious consciousness, owe much to the character of the *milieu* within which the child is brought up. The various stages of this development cannot be described in any strictly chronological sequence because the child's growing awareness of himself as an entity distinct from his family, and his curiosity about the 'how' and the 'why' of life, develop so rapidly that they appear almost simultaneously. The most important single influence in the child's earliest development is exercised by his parents: 'When we endeavour to formulate the child's ideas of his father and mother, we find them to include the divine attributes of classical theology: omnipotence,

[1] Henri Clavier: *L'Idée de Dieu chez l'Enfant*: p. 14, quoted B. A. Yeaxlee: *Religion and the Growing Mind* (1945) pp. 39–40.

omniscience and moral perfection.'[1] Freud argued, as we have seen, that the young child comes to his ideas of God as the result of his unconscious appreciation of the part played in his life by his parents, so that 'God is at bottom nothing but an exalted father'.[2] This implies that adult belief in God is nothing more than a projection continued from childhood. But there are two cogent objections to such a conclusion.

It could be argued, from the Jungian point of view, that the child comes to regard his father as the God-imago because of the operation of the God-archetype, or, as Professor L. Binswanger stated it (without referring to the possible existence of the God-archetype), 'the fact that the child is receptive to the child-father idea is the result of the typically ideal existence of the child-father idea born of our relation to God'.[3] The second objection has been well stated by Canon L. W. Grensted:

> The mechanism of which Freud speaks . . . is a perfectly real process within the reality of the ego itself. It is essential to the whole theory of projection that the transferred and dissociated affects are attracted to some perfectly real object which is significant for the ego in some way. We do not cast our shadow-gods out upon a void. The ego never creates entities. There is always an objective basis upon which the fantasy rests.[4]

This point is reinforced by Dr Ruth Griffiths who says that in the years between say three and seven, the child is influenced by his imaginative processes, the development of which leads to a series of phantastical projections because 'phantasy is the means by which the child overcomes his environment, learns gradually to face reality and brings about his development'.[5] It is unrealistic to say that because the child uses the 'picture-language of phantasy' there is no external reality that awakens these feelings of wonder and awe within. The young child like primitive man is aware of Something which arouses in him a feeling of wonder and mystery.[6] 'Impulse and appetite and

[1] Pierre Bovet: *Le Sentiment Religieux et la Psychologie de l'Infant*: Eng. trans. G. H. Green: *The Child's Religion* (1928) p. 30.

[2] Freud: *Totem and Taboo*: p. 225.

[3] Quoted by H. C. Rümke: *The Psychology of Unbelief* (1952) p. 30.

[4] L. W. Grensted: *Psychology and God* (1930) p. 64.

[5] Ruth Griffiths: *Imagination in Early Childhood* (1935) p. 11.

[6] McDougall has pointed out that every instinct is *teleologically* directed. Man's instinctual striving towards a goal is something more than a biological process, since it can involve the apprehension of some object about which man formulates a sentiment which may be described as 'religious'. The hormic nature of instinctual and emotional activities may be interpreted philosophically as indicating that the

emotion and sentiment only have meaning in a world to which they are successively appropriate. Hunger would be as meaningless in a foodless world as sex would be in a world where we were not organized as men and women.' [1] That this sense of reality cannot be entertained by the young child independently of personal relationships is due to the fact that the child's early development takes place within a strongly personal environment. But as the child grows older and reaches the age of six or seven, he arrives at that stage of realism where he feels the need to turn to a wider and more varied environment than that of the immediate family.[2] The child now becomes interested in the 'scientific' picture of the world, which is accompanied by what may be called an 'embryonic interest in metaphysics', for the child is interested not only in the scientific How? but also in the philosophical Why? This coincides with the child's developing religious and social sense, a development which often brings him into conflict with parental views. Edmund Gosse gives a vivid example of an experience which occurred somewhere between his sixth and seventh birthdays. His father, who was a Plymouth Brother, had been speaking about the idolatry of 'heathen religions'.

> I cross-examined my Father very closely as to the nature of this sin, and pinned him down to the categorical statement that idolatry consisted in praying to any one or anything but God Himself. Wood and stone, in the words of the hymn, were peculiarly liable to be bowed down to by the heathen in their blindness . . . my Father assured me that God would be very angry and would signify His anger, if any one in a Christian country, bowed down to wood and stone.

The young boy, however, determined to put the matter to the test.

> I was in the morning-room on the ground-floor, where with much labour, I hoisted a small chair on the table close to the window. My heart was now beating as if it would leap out of my side, but I pursued my experiment. I knelt down on the carpet in front of the table and looking up I said my daily prayer in a loud voice, only substituting the address, 'O Chair!' for the habitual one.

Nothing happened, even though it was a fine day, 'there was not a cloud in the sky, not an unusual sound in the street. Presently I was quite sure that nothing would happen. I had committed idolatry,

---

child's impulses are directed not to some infantile phantasy but to some objective reality.

[1] L. W. Grensted: *This Business of Living* (1939) p. 82.

[2] See Susan Isaacs: *Intellectual Growth in Young Children* (1930).

flagrantly and deliberately, and God did not care.' [1] The result was not any diminution of the boy's belief in God, but of his father's understanding of the nature of idolatry!

As puberty approaches the earlier interest in rational queries seems for a time to be displaced either by a return to the earlier non-rational stages, or, more frequently, by an advance to some supra-rational interest. It is at this stage that the child often has his first religious experience. Not only does his awareness of an external environment give rise to a religiously interrogative attitude, it also increases the number of situations which evoke fear. This is what we should expect. The imaginative life of primitive man is similarly associated with strong emotions of fear arising from situations which are dangerous, taboo or sacred. This sense of fear is not only part of the developing religious consciousness of the child, it is also part of his developing moral sense, for religion and morality develop within the same context.

The Child's Moral Sense

The young child gains his first standards of behaviour from the teaching of his parents and other grown-up persons. If he observes a discrepancy between their teaching and their behaviour this gives rise to doubt and perplexity which if carried into adolescence may furnish a partial explanation of much that is described as juvenile delinquency.

Freud's concept of the Super-Ego has provided an explanation of the origin of man's moral ideals. The Super-Ego deals with the Ego rather as a strict father deals with his child, and assumes the status of 'conscience'. Melanie Klein, discussing the early development of conscience in the child,[2] says that 'the conscience is a precipitate or representation of his early relations with his parents'. In the course of her analysis of children under four years of age, she found that their Super-Egos were harsher and more cruel than those of their parents, and harsher than those of older children. This seems to indicate that conscience should not, therefore, be totally identified with the Super-Ego. A more acceptable explanation of conscience is that offered by Dr J. A. Hadfield who advanced the view that conscience involves the same psychological processes as temptation. 'Temptation is the voice of the suppressed evil when the good is dominant, and conscience is

[1] Edmund Gosse: *Father and Son*: Evergreen Books edn (1941) pp. 43–4.

[2] See Melanie Klein: *Contributions to Psycho-Analysis – 1921–1945* (1948) pp. 267 ff.

the voice of the suppressed good when evil is dominant.' [1] How far the behaviour of the young child is determined by conscience or the Super-Ego is not clear. Conscience in the strict sense of the word involves a consciousness of sin, but 'sin' for the young is often nothing more than a refusal to obey a parental order.

The moral sense begins to operate more clearly about the stage of puberty and gives rise to an accompanying sense of guilt. Sin and guilt are inextricably associated, but how far this is a natural development or how far it is a 'religious imposition' it is difficult to decide. Evangelical Christianity has been particularly insistent that the young should be brought under the conviction of sin, a process which has caused many children to develop an exaggerated sense of guilt between the ages of seven and twelve. During these years the child adds to the standards of the family, the code of the 'club' or the 'gang'. This, during adolescence, is to some extent replaced by the conscious acceptance of more strictly moral standards. At the same time, the adolescent under the pressure, praise, criticism and encouragement of family, school, sports club and church reaches a clearer picture of how he *ought* to behave.[2] External standards are interiorized and identified with the inherent possibilities of a youth's own nature, so that the adolescent begins to arrive at the stage of a morally responsible person; but this does not necessarily involve the recognition of a universal ethical standard unless the social and religious environments are favourable.

Adolescence and Conversion

Ever since Starbuck wrote *The Psychology of Religion* (1899) it has been agreed that the adolescent sense of sin is also accompanied by the growth of altruistic sentiments. The adolescent sense of sin in previous generations (though markedly less so today) in many cases arose from an almost morbid adult insistence upon the sinfulness of sex.[3] It is true that adolescence often comes to a climax in 'conversion' but this 'conversion' is not necessarily of a moral character. Conversion is a term that can be applied to particular stages in the

[1] J. A. Hadfield: *Psychology and Morals* (London) 1925: pp. 37 ff.

[2] P. Nunn: *Education: Its Data and First Principles* (1941) pp. 174 ff.

[3] More than a hundred years ago, Emerson protested that 'Our young people are diseased with the theological problems of original sin, origin of evil, predestination and the like. These never darkened across any man's road who did not go out of his way to seek them. These are the soul's mumps, and measles, and whooping-coughs.' Emerson: *Spiritual Laws*, quoted James: *Varieties*: p. 167 n.

social, aesthetic and religious development of the adolescent, if by it we mean 'the achievement of a new or unified personality' as the result of a reorientation of the psyche to some new ideal or purpose. It is often assumed that all such events are sudden and dramatic irruptions into the ordinary level of consciousness, but this fails to allow for the slow and concealed processes of the unconscious whose climaxes may appear as sudden decisions but are really the long-prepared-for results of unconscious 'incubation'.

As an example of the protracted results of a moral experience which occurred at an early age, developed into a painful moral problem during adolescence and came to a brave religious decision in adulthood, we may quote George Borrow's famous account of the experience of Peter Williams, the Welsh preacher:

> I was born in the heart of North Wales, the son of a respectable farmer, and am the youngest of seven brothers.
>
> My father was a member of the Church of England, and was what is generally called a serious man. He went to church regularly, and read the Bible every Sunday evening; in his moments of leisure he was fond of holding religious discourse both with his family and his neighbours. . . .

Peter, who was then about seven years old, one evening heard his father and a neighbour discussing the 'sin against the Holy Ghost'.

> 'Ah! said my father, 'thank God I never committed that – how awful must be the state of a person who has committed the sin against the Holy Ghost! I can scarcely think of it without my hair standing on end;' and then my father and his friend began talking of the nature of the sin against the Holy Ghost, and I heard them say what it was, as I sat with greedy ears listening to their discourse.
>
> I lay awake the greater part of the night musing upon what I had heard. . . . Once or twice I felt a strong inclination to commit it, a strange sense of fear, however, prevented me. . . .
>
> When I awoke in the morning the first thing I thought of was the mysterious sin, and a voice within me seemed to say, 'Commit it', and I felt a strong temptation to do so, even stronger than in the night . . . [but] springing out of bed, I went down on my knees. I slept in a small room alone, to which I ascended by a wooden stair, open to the sky. . . .

An interval elapsed, but waking one night the young boy determined that nothing should prevent him from committing the sin.

> Arising from my bed, I went out upon the wooden gallery; and having stood for a few moments looking at the stars, with which the heavens were thickly strewn, I laid myself down, and supporting my face with my hand, I murmured out words of horror – words not to be repeated, and in this manner I committed the sin against the Holy Ghost.

> When the words were uttered I sat up upon the topmost step of the gallery; for some time I felt stunned in somewhat the same manner as I once subsequently felt after being stung by an adder. . . .

Time went by and Peter made great progress at school, but always with a sense of being separated from his school-fellows by a great gulf. Then his father fell ill and shortly afterwards, feeling that death was near, called for his children and after embracing them said:

> 'God bless you, my children; I am going from you, but take comfort, I trust that we shall all meet again in heaven.'
>
> As he uttered these last words, horror took entire possession of me. Meet my father in heaven – how could I ever hope to meet him there? . . . In a few days my father died: . . . I still remained at school . . . I was diligent both in self-improvement and in the instruction of others; nevertheless a horrible weight pressed upon my breast; I knew I was a lost being; that for me there was no hope . . . I had committed the unpardonable sin, for which I was doomed to eternal punishment, in the flaming gulf, as soon as life was over!

Still more time elapsed. A certain element of religious joy filled his life for a time as the result of a brief experience one fine morning as he was at work in the fields, but the dreadful and horrifying sense of guilt increased with the years. It persisted through his married life until one day he met a young man who impressed upon him that the experience by which his soul was harrowed was of frequent occurrence among children, and this was one of the means by which God 'had permitted him to be chastened for a season', that his lamp might burn the brighter for all that he had undergone.[1] It is obvious that here we have an account of long unhappy years of guilt and remorse leading to a final sense of redemption in late life, a protracted experience that was due to a heavily laden theological environment in childhood. But the more normal and conventional forms of conversion are those of individuals who, becoming aware of interior conflicts, feel an urgent sense of the need for reformation – a feeling that is often accompanied by disturbingly strong emotions.

The more emotional of these experiences occur in personalities whom James described as 'twice-born'.[2] The twice-born exhibit a marked discord in their native temperament, a discrepancy between their religious convictions and their temperamental constitution.

[1] George Borrow: *Lavengro*: chaps. 75–79.

[2] This distinction between the once-born and the twice-born was derived from F. W. Newman's *The Soul: Its Sorrows and its Aspirations* (1852 edn) pp. 89 ff. 'God has two families of children on this earth, the once-born and the twice-born.'

The comparatively undisturbed moral consciousness of the once-born causes the twice-born to regard them as persons whose lives are lacking in religious depth. Upon this William James made the pertinent observation that

> the final consciousness which each type reaches of union with the divine has the same practical significance for the individual: and individuals may well be allowed to get to it by the channels which lie open to their several temperaments . . . [so that] in many cases it is quite arbitrary whether we class the individual as a once-born or a twice-born subject.[1]

Adolescence and Religion

The reassuring protection of his parents is essential to the young child's development, but the adolescent seeks a wider circle of encouragement. He needs a companion and a confidant who is able to arouse in him that element of hero-worship which later will enable him to achieve the highest of all sentiments, reverence. If this companion is a somewhat older person and religious then the result can be highly beneficial to the adolescent. An illuminating example is provided by the experience of a boy of twelve:

> The vicar visited my parents and persuaded them to let me be confirmed as soon as I was twelve. He founded a scout troop, and I joined it. Meanwhile, another man had come upon the scene, the vicar's friend B., who became curate and assistant scout-master – he it was who paid for my uniform which my parents could not afford to buy. He coached us in a religious phantasia that the vicar (Captain) was arranging. The influence of the Captain and of B. was inestimable. I was confirmed; between them they tried to change the church from extremely Low Church to Anglo-Catholic – they instructed me in their creed, and as the change came about so my interest in religion became an obsession. I was thrilled when asked to be a server at Holy Communion. I would get up any morning of the week to serve for Captain when he especially asked me . . . B. took me to London in his car on All Saints's Day to the High Mass service at All Saints' Church, Margaret Street. It was my first introduction to the use of incense which, when wafted over the church, intoxicated me. A further way in which B. influenced me and made me realise the all-pervading spirit of God was when he, in the privacy of his own room, talked to me on the problems of sex, explaining in the most beautiful manner everything that, up to that time, like most boys from eight to thirteen, I had found out from the wrong sources. The whole subject now seemed to reveal to me God in yet another sphere.[2]

---

[1] James: *Varieties*: p. 488.

[2] Margaret Phillips: *The Education of the Emotions through Sentiment Development* (1937) pp. 265–6.

But the sense of religion is seriously affected in late adolescence if the young person is involved, as frequently happens, in an emotional situation arising from disappointment or loneliness. Here is the case of an adolescent girl who had lost her friend, developed a rather sentimental attachment to religion, and then herself falling in love experienced a decline in religious interest.

> Because I was lonely, now that my friend had become engaged, I went to another church and enjoyed myself emotionally by having a crush on the vicar. My literature now was almost solely religious. I read the *Imitation*, the *Garden of the Soul*, the *Breviary*, and every book of Catholic devotion upon which I could lay my hands. . . . By Easter, I discovered I was in love and that life had become more complex. I was still continuing churchgoing, in fact, my going off to Lenten watches before the Blessed Sacrament had caused a quarrel. But the enthusiasm was dying. When I should have been thinking holy thoughts I was longing for the service to be over, so that I might meet him outside.[1]

It is clear that for many the changes from childhood to adolescence and from adolescence to adulthood are often periods of 'storm and stress' but it is a mistake to treat these experiences as being exclusively moral or religious. To restrict adolescent crises too exclusively to moral difficulties is to obscure the fact that many a conversion crisis is really an intellectual dilemma.[2] Conversely, an intellectual problem may sometimes prove to be a theological disguise for a moral difficulty. It is a common experience for a practising psychiatrist, or a priest acting as a confessor, to hear a young adult saying that he cannot believe any longer in such a childish superstition as the existence of God. Such a statement, however, is sometimes an intellectual disguise for a suppressed sense of sin and guilt. If God could be dismissed from our personal universe, then for many people there would be no such thing as sin and no feeling of guilt. In late adolescence, and more particularly in adulthood, conversions of an intellectual kind can and do occur without any sense of moral guilt. Pratt gives two lengthy instances drawn, first, from Max Müller's *Life and Sayings of Ramakrishna*[3] and, secondly, from the life of Maharshi.

[1] Margaret Phillips: op. cit. pp. 274–5.

[2] Doubt should be distinguished from mere scepticism. Doubt indicates a deep concern about spiritual interpretations of the universe. Jacques Maritain says that atheists and agnostics may in their doubt be choosing God as the true object of their lives' devotion; while Paul Tillich says that 'God who is absent as the object of faith is present as the source of that restlessness which asks ultimate questions about the meaning of life'.

[3] J. B. Pratt: *The Religious Consciousness* (1930) pp. 129 ff.

Devendranath Tagore, the father of the famous Bengalee poet, Rabindranath Tagore.[1]

Ramakrishna (b. 1833) belonged to a poor but high-caste Brahmin family, and from his boyhood was intensely religious. At the age of eleven he had a vision at the sight of white cranes flying against the brilliant blue of the Indian sky. At twenty, he began to frequent the shrines of the Mother Goddess, Kali. We are told that for years the young Ramakrishna, who had a very strong sense of caste, would weep because the Mother Goddess did not reveal herself to him as completely as he yearned for. It is clear, says Pratt, that the young Ramakrishna was 'a divided personality' but there was very little of the 'storm and stress' of adolescent sexuality in his life, his preoccupation for some twelve years was with this ideal to which he sought to direct his attention. At last he came to realize, as the result of a religious experience, that he could not know his ideal – the Mother Goddess – unless he gave up 'the love of his little self'.[2] From this time onwards he came to believe that 'the sense of "I" in us is the greatest obstacle in the path of God-vision. It covers the Truth. When "I" is dead, all trouble ceases.' In other words, as the result of intellectual illumination, Ramakrishna achieved by a surrender of self that integration of personality in which moral, emotional and intellectual harmony became an established fact and left him free to seek without further hindrance his great ideal – the Mother Goddess.

In the second case, young Tagore, brought up in a rich and ortho-

[1] J. B. Pratt: op. cit. pp. 133 ff., and the *Autobiography of Maharshi Devendranath Tagore.*

[2] This sense of the need to give up 'the love of the little self' forms part of the psychological structure of conversions in many religions. Dr R. H. Thouless, commenting on the conversion of William Booth, the founder of the Salvation Army (see Harold Begbie: *Life of William Booth*: 2 vols. 1920), says that Booth as a boy was overshadowed by the financial difficulties of his family and the fact that very early on he was sent to work in a pawnbroker's shop. This humiliating experience, his father's death and his sense of the social evils of his time, not only increased his adolescent unhappiness but deepened his sense of his need for God. As a boy he had managed to make a profit out of a companion by a trick the memory of which lay heavily on his conscience. He found that he could not bring himself to God until he had broken the façade of his personal probity by a confession of his boyish sin. 'In his sixteenth year, he determined to make *the surrender of personality* which precedes conversion.' R. H. Thouless: *An Introduction to the Psychology of Religion* (1936) p. 218. This he managed to do by a sudden confession to the person whom he had deceived. Here we have another instance of the fact that conversion, whether it includes a sense of guilt or not, always involves this feeling of need to give up this 'love of the little self' before one can achieve that re-orientation which is a turning of oneself to another Goal.

dox family, found that his family's worship of Kali and Vishnu sufficed until his eighteenth year when, upon the death of his grandmother, he experienced a 'spontaneous awakening'. This passed, to be succeeded by a period of spiritual depression and despair. His despair was not caused by any sense of moral guilt, but by a sense of *spiritual ignorance*. 'He wanted insight, he wanted relief from the weary weight of all this unintelligible world.' But intellectual difficulties in religion are never purely intellectual. What the seeker needs most of all is not a translucent explanation of the mystery of the universe but some absolutely convincing Object to which he can direct his life and at the same time feel himself irresistibly drawn. In other words, the young Tagore was vividly conscious of an *incompleteness* which needed some *metaphysical* solution that would provide 'a new centre of loyalty'.

At first sight, these examples of religious development may seem to be strangely different from the examples quoted earlier on. The experiences of a youngster whose religious development was helped by the friendly encouragement of a young clergyman (*his* confidant), and a young girl whose religious interests were plainly related to her emotional attachments, seem to be quite different from those of two personalities who from their earliest years were surrounded by a highly developed religious atmosphere. Yet in all of these cases, there is a common pattern. The young, as they become conscious of a greater world than that of their immediate family, become aware of the need of some purpose that will give them '*something to live for*'. This is a normal pattern of religious development and it need not be accompanied by any feeling of moral guilt (though in many cases it is) nor yet by periods of storm-and-stress. All men – and this is one of the facts which Freud seems never to have discussed – in their desire for 'completeness' exhibit some form (however confused and unrealized) of metaphysical interest. The 'How' of life is always accompanied by the 'Why' of existence, and this is convincingly furnished for every young man and woman for whom some Person, Object or End is suddenly or gradually revealed as *the real purpose of life*. Whether this be described as a religious experience, a revelation or a conversion, is quite immaterial, the result in all cases is the same – 'a new man'.

We can illustrate this by a typical example of the sort of conversion achieved in the early days of the Oxford Group (Moral Rearmament) Movement. Three young women spent a day in Oxford with some undergraduate friends. One of them describes her experiences as follows:

> We had a great day at Oxford and were introduced to about eight or nine of Hugh's friends, men and women, who throughout our day there showed the most wonderful and sympathetic attitude towards us. Their conduct was a revelation. I have never known such a spirit and companionship in its most Christ-like sense. . . . The climax of the whole day was when we returned to Hugh's rooms for coffee. As I believe now, it was all a part of God's good plan for me that I should have had the opportunity of a private conversation with Mary . . . she had absolutely given herself to God, and now firmly believed that she was working under God's guidance. I could see, as she progressed, that she was living with and on something that did give a tremendous zest to life. Through the Oxford Group she had found Christianity in its practical sense, which was helping her to live life abundantly, so that the mere material troubles of life, exams, money, what people thought of her, her own well-being, everything that most of us value above all things, formed no place in her life. My other two friends, luckily were of the same mind, and in the train on the way home we all thought of life with God, and not ourselves, as the centre.[1]

Here again, we see the same impulse at work. If in previous generations, adolescents and young adults were often induced to believe that they must, as a primary condition of a religious life, experience a highly emotional moral conversion, today conversion assumes a new variation of an old form. This is true whether we are dealing with the intellectual difficulties of orientals, with undergraduates, young boy-scouts or girls in love. The basic pattern of religious experience is the same everywhere, no matter how different the superstructure may be – a matter that will engage our attention in a later chapter.

[1] Margaret Phillips: op. cit. pp. 279–80.

Chapter IX

THE PSYCHOLOGY OF RELIGIOUS PRACTICES – PRAYER

If we ask what are the psychical functions of religion, the answer is three-fold. First, religion is that which enables man to satisfy certain non-physical needs; secondly, it is that which results from experiences which involve the active participation of the supra-personal forces of the unconscious; and, thirdly, it is an activity which assumes common forms in different types of religion. Two of the most important of these activities are Prayer and Worship, which are so closely related that one cannot be discussed without the other. Yet despite the closeness of their relationship, there are distinctive aspects such as make it necessary to consider them separately.

* * *

Prayer – Definitions and Kinds

In one of the most comprehensive studies of Prayer, Professor Friedrich Heiler[1] described prayer as

> the spontaneous expression of upspringing religious experiences, and as the mechanical recitation of an incomprehensible formula . . . as the involuntary discharge of an overwhelming emotion, and as the voluntary concentration on a religious object: . . . as loud shouting and crying, and as still, silent absorption . . . as joyous thanksgiving and as ecstatic praise, and as humble supplication for forgiveness and compassion . . . as a simple petition for daily bread, and as an all-consuming yearning for God himself . . . as a stormy clamour and demand, and as joyful renunciation and holy serenity: as a desire to change God's will and make it chime with our petty wishes, and as a self-forgetting vision of and surrender to the Highest Good . . . as the trustful talk of a child with a kind father: as the humble petition of a servant to a powerful master, and as the ecstatic converse of the bride with the heavenly Bridegroom.[2]

[1] Friedrich Heiler: *Prayer: A Study in the History and Psychology of Religion* (1932) Eng. trans.

[2] op. cit. p. 353.

If this description of the many forms in which prayer can be offered seems to be too inclusive it is because we are apt to forget that religion is so closely allied with the totality of life that there is no aspect of human experience which is not its direct concern. But prayer is not merely a psychological activity, though as a human engagement it calls for a psychological explanation; nor is it something that begins and ends with the human voice –

> *. . . prayer is more*
> *Than an order of words, the conscious occupation*
> *Of the praying mind, or the sound of the voice praying . . .*[1]

Or, as Archbishop Söderblom has expressed it: 'in prayer we have not a mere echo of our own voice, of our own being, resounding from the dark depths of personality, but a reality higher and greater than our own, which we can adore and in which we trust'.[2] Prayer in essence is 'a living communion of the religious man with God, conceived as personal and present in experience, a communion which reflects the forms of the social relations of humanity . . .'[3] The psychological nature of prayer can be arrived at only by studying it from various standpoints, and here again – as in our discussion of the origins of religion – we have first to consider prayer in its more primitive forms.

Prayer and Primitive Man

Studies of the prayerful attitudes of primitive man are psychologically of considerable importance since they indicate the basic motives behind this activity. Modern studies have made it clear that the individual does not emerge from the group mind until comparatively late in the history of human development, so that the prayers of primitive people tend to be in the nature of group utterances. This suggests that the oldest forms of prayer are the collective cries of the group, or silent participation on the part of the tribe in the prayers offered for the tribe by its leader. We may suppose that such prayers, implying some recognition of the supernatural, began with an invocation followed it may be by a complaint protesting vehemently against some catastrophe, cruelty or frustration. But it is petition rather than complaint that is the core of prayer. Man normally prays *for* something related to his well-being, whether this be for preservation from danger, or for increase of children, food, flocks or crops.

[1] T. S. Eliot: *Little Gidding* (*Four Quartets*).
[2] Söderblom, quoted Heiler: op. cit. p. 358. [3] idem.

This element of undisguised self-interest is in itself indicative of one of the underlying motives of prayer. Even in the more developed forms of religion, in the Rig-Veda for instance, the materialistic nature of primitive prayer continues so that in the later religions of antiquity, East and West, prayers are largely embellished forms of primitive petition. Such prayers were usually offered with a gift. Prayer and sacrifice develop together. Even if we do not accept Freud's totemic explanation of the origin of sacrificial religion (which we shall discuss later), it would appear that the act of sacrifice formed part of the group's petitionary approach to the tribal deity at certain stages of development. This sacrificial act may be interpreted either as one of propitiation, or else as an act of thanksgiving and praise which becomes a form of worship. Gestures such as standing to pray with head bowed and arms folded, kneeling or lying prostrate, the lifting up of hands either as an invocatory gesture or as an apotropaic movement, were originally spontaneous and dramatic accompaniments of petitionary prayer in one form or another.[1] That these gestures remain to the present day in all kinds of religion, even if in a highly formalized manner, is evidence both of their natural origin and of the power of habit and group suggestion.

It is necessary to add only a brief note about primitive man's concept of the supernatural as we have already discussed this earlier on. The supernatural for primitive man is closely associated with objects thought of as possessing *mana* or endowed with a life of the same kind as that of the worshippers themselves. This explains why primitive man in his prayers believed that he could persuade his god to change his mind in the petitioner's favour. This sense of kinship between the mind of the petitioner and that of his god assumed in the course of religious development a mystical character in the prayer-life of the great religions of the world.

Motives

If it be asked 'why do men pray?' the answer is that there is no one single motive. Prayer psychologically involves not only a sense of material need, it also involves a psychical hunger for some higher form of life.

> The hungry pygmy who begs for food, the entranced mystic absorbed in the greatness and beauty of the infinite God, the guilt oppressed

[1] 'Let the lifting up of my hands be an evening sacrifice', Ps. cxli. 2, refers to the part played by gesture and the association of sacrifice and prayer.

> Christian who prays for forgiveness of sins and assurance of salvation . . . all are seeking a confirmation and an enrichment of their realization of life.[1]

To which we have to add the affirmation that 'the effort to fortify, to reinforce, to enhance one's life' is one of the motives in all forms of prayer. Such an effort involves a deliberate turning of the psyche to the transcendental and the divine. 'The human heart is as sensitive to God as the retina is to light waves. The soul possesses a native yearning for intercourse and companionship which takes it to God as naturally as the homing instinct of the pigeon takes it to the place of its birth.' [2] But we must be careful not to suggest that man has an *instinct* to pray – man has a need for 'completeness' which is the master sentiment in a hierarchy of sentiments. The Law of Completeness operates in all aspects of man's religious life and not least of all in his prayerful activities. This feeling of need for completeness must not be interpreted as being purely subjective. Man could not experience hunger if there had never been the objective means of satisfying that hunger. Prayer, psychologically, is one of the many aspects of the soul's need for completeness. According to William James, we pray because we cannot help praying.[3] This statement, for James, depends upon the conviction that man by experience learns that he is 'continuous' with a Greater Self from whom all experience in religion is derived, and to whom man is drawn as are iron filings to a magnet. It is certain that one of the motives of prayer is the impulse to converse with the Divine, an impulse which is the subject of philosophical exposition in Martin Buber's discussion of the I–Thou relationship.[4]

This need to pray in the sense of seeking communion with the Divine is indigenous to every religion, rises spontaneously in men at all levels of culture and forms a basic impulse in religion of all kinds.

> There is something in the structure of the soul, in the nature of personal self-consciousness which prepares the way for mystic vision which fits us for [that] type of experience. . . . We are framed and made for intercourse with a supersensuous world and we cannot live within the limits of the tangible and describable world.[5]

---

[1] Heiler: op. cit. p. 355.

[2] Rufus Jones: 'Prayer and the Mystic Vision': in *Concerning Prayer* (1931) ed. B. H. Streeter: p. 118.

[3] William James: *Principles of Psychology*: Vol. I. p. 316.

[4] Martin Buber: *I and Thou* (1937).

[5] Rufus Jones: op. cit. pp. 108–9.

This agrees with the views of one of the earliest of the Greek Fathers, Clement of Alexandria (fl. A.D. 210), who said that there is something in the very nature of man which makes him a religious being capable of 'that divine and mutual reciprocal correspondence' which is the essence of prayer. These views support the belief that prayer is not a monologue, that it is a conversation, a listening and a response; the expression of a need to speak of one's self, one's needs, aspirations, fears and gratitude to some other Self than man's egocentric personality – and to await a reply. But this conclusion has to face the criticism that such 'conversations' may after all be nothing more than a form of auto-suggestion, the self speaking about the self to the self.

Prayer and Auto-Suggestion

Since it is sometimes affirmed that prayer is nothing but a form of auto-suggestion it is important to see what such a statement implies. Suggestion is generally defined as a mental process which leads to the uncritical acceptance by one person of ideas from another person, an acceptance which finally issues in action or belief. Auto-suggestion is another name for self-suggestion, but what is called *auto*-suggestion may in fact be a disguised form of *hetero*-suggestion. The relationship of suggestion to prayer arises from a distinction made by Baudouin between *spontaneous* and *reflective* forms of auto-suggestion.[1] Spontaneous suggestion is the result of something that catches the subject's attention as it were inadvertently. Reflective suggestion arises from a subject's deliberate concentration of his attention upon some specific idea or situation. This concentration can sometimes be achieved by using some such simple technique as repeating many times a short phrase expressive of a particular idea upon which the subject wishes to steady his attention.[2] The use of such techniques of concentration seems to lend support to the critical

[1] Charles Baudouin: *Suggestion and Auto-suggestion* (1920) pp. 116 ff.

[2] Such a method was practised by the followers of al-Ghazzali: 'Let the seeker . . . sit alone in some corner, limiting his religious duties to what are absolutely incumbent . . . let him see to it that nothing save God most High enters his mind. Then as he sits alone . . . let him not cease saying continuously with his tongue, "Allah, Allah," keeping his thought on it. At last he will reach a state where the motion of his tongue will cease, and it will seem as though the word flowed from it. Let him persevere in this until all form of the word is removed from his tongue . . . until the form of the word is removed from his heart, and there remains the idea alone as though clinging to his heart, inseparable from it. . . . Nothing now remains, but to wait what God will open to him. . . .' Quoted by Macdonald: *Religious Attitude and Life in Islam* (1909) pp. 255–6: cited by J. B. Pratt: op. cit. p. 390 n.

comment that prayer is auto-suggestive and purely subjective. But prayer is not a subjective exercise – it is a conversation. Canon Grensted, commenting on prayer and auto-suggestion, says:

> The criticism . . . that we are really addressing ourselves, drawing our assurances from tradition and from many other sources, and simply using auto-suggestion . . . is very often true. . . . But even so it should be noted that such auto-suggestion rests upon a prior suggestion from outside. The first impulse to pray does not arise from within. It has in fact a twofold origin. The first prayers of the child are taught by, and are said to, the mother or teacher. . . . There is no auto-suggestion about this at all. It is simply vocal intercourse turned in a particular direction. It becomes prayer when the child begins to realize that it is not speaking to its mother, but with its mother to that which lies beyond. Vocal prayer, the simplest and most direct form of prayer, is thus the most natural and in the end the highest. . . . The real advance in prayer comes not with increased complexity in such exercises but in the growing assurance of the reality of God who hears us and responds.[1]

This straightforward exposition of the two-way nature of prayer makes it clear that prayer is a natural expression of the psyche (as natural and as paternally trained as speech itself) and that it is not a purely subjective form of suggestion. The various techniques employed to produce a state of concentration, or an emptiness of mind,[2] that leaves the subject open to a divine suggestion, vary from such comfortable and relaxed physical methods as those outlined by Baudouin[3] to the physically trained postures (*asana*) of the Yogin who achieve a release from external intrusions by a posture that produces an almost hypnoidal condition. But a theological difference introduces itself at this point into any discussion of prayerful techniques. Prayer, from the Christian point of view, is 'the hour when the continual presence of the awful Sovereign of the creature is, in a certain sense, made actual and real, when the heart speaks to God, and what is of infinitely greater moment – when God speaks to the heart'.[4] But Indian religions, as well as other mystical types of reli-

[1] L. W. Grensted: *The Psychology of Religion* (1952) pp. 126–7.

[2] Auto-suggestion applies not to prayer itself but only to some of the techniques which are laid down in various manuals of instruction. See, for instance, Fr Bede Frost: *The Art of Mental Prayer* (1932) pp. 49–132, for an account of the Ignatian, Franciscan, Carmelite, Salesian, Liguorian and Oratorian methods. This book contains a valuable Bibliography. Another highly useful book with a good Bibliography is Fr Hubert Northcott C.R.: *The Venture of Prayer* (1951). The author is indebted to both of these works.

[3] op. cit.

[4] Bishop Hedley: quoted by Fr Bede Frost: *The Art of Mental Prayer* (1932) p. 46. See also Dom Cuthbert Butler O.S.B., *Western Mysticism* (1926), Grey Arrow edn (1960) pp. 21 ff., for 'Bishop Hedley on Contemplation'.

gion, are concerned mainly with the achieving of union with the Eternal rather than with eliciting a reply from deity. It is this aspect of prayer which relates it closely to the general pattern of mysticism.

Prayer and Mysticism

Mystical prayer, which is sometimes described as 'contemplative prayer', is distinguished from other forms of prayer because it often begins and ends without any apparent effort on the part of the person praying.[1] Mme Guyon refers to this kind of prayer when she says:

> What surprised me most is that I had great difficulty in saying my spoken prayers which I had been in the custom of saying. As soon as I opened my mouth to pronounce them the [divine] love seized me so strongly that I remained absorbed in profound silence and in a peace which I cannot express.[2]

Prayers of this kind cannot be described as petitionary nor yet as verbal conversations; petitionary elements are present in such prayers only if they are of the kind that St Augustine refers to when he says 'Ask nothing from God except God himself.' It is a form of prayer which has such a small place for words that it has been compared by St François de Sales to the 'communion' of lovers: 'Love speaks not merely by the tongue, but by the eyes, the posture, the sighs: yes, even silence takes the place of words.' [3] But silence and the absence of words are not restricted to mystical prayer only. They are part of the

[1] St Bernard of Clairvaux declared: 'I confess, then, to speak foolishly, that the Word has visited me – indeed, very often. But, though He has frequently come into my soul, I have never at any time been aware of the moment of His coming. I have felt Him present, I remember He has been with me, I have sometimes even had a premonition of His coming, but never have I felt His coming or departure. . . . It is not by the eyes that He enters, for He has no colour; nor by the ears for His coming is silent: nor by the nostrils for He is blended with the mind, and not with the air; nor again does He enter by the mouth, for His nature cannot be eaten or drunk; nor lastly can we trace Him by touch, for He is intangible. You will ask me then how, since His track is thus trackless, I could know that He is present? Because He is living and full of energy, and as soon as He has entered me, has quickened my sleeping soul, and aroused, softened and goaded my heart which was torpid and hard as stone. . . . In the reformation and renewal of the spirit of my mind, that is my inward man, I have seen something of the loveliness of His Beauty, and meditating on these things have been filled with wonder at the multitude of His greatness. But when the Word withdrew, all these spiritual powers and faculties began to droop and languish, as if the fire were taken from beneath a bubbling pot; and this is to me the sign of His departure.' St Bernard of Clairvaux: *Canticles*: quoted by Evelyn Underhill: *The Mystics of the Church* (1925) pp. 86–7.

[2] Mme Guyon: quoted by Segond in *La Prière*, p. 185.

[3] Quoted by Pratt: op. cit. p. 328.

general technique of such forms of group prayer as are commonly observed by the members of the Society of Friends, where a 'mutual lending out of our minds' creates an atmosphere from which the intrusive elements of daily life are excluded in favour of a silent approach to the supernatural.[1] Mystical prayer, therefore, is virtually indistinguishable from mystical experience; both include an interior feeling of relationship with an invisible reality such as raises the life of the experient to its highest level of unity and integration. What then are the chief psychological characteristics of mystical prayer?

We have already noted that such prayer involves a deliberate concentration of attention, and the employment of techniques of preparation which are sometimes subject to sudden intrusions from the unconscious. Compared with the emotional quality of spontaneous outbursts of vocal prayer which express needs and desires, mystical prayer is one which subjects all feelings and sensations to an act of aspiration so that, to quote St Thomas Aquinas, mystical prayer is 'the ascent of the mind to God', it is the prayer of the ladder. But how is this concentration achieved? Most authorities decide that it involves at least three elements: (*a*) the *purgative*, as the means of detachment from the everyday world,[2] (*b*) the *illuminative*, by which the soul seeks for peace and fervent love, and (*c*) the *unitive* way, in which the soul is conscious of the presence of God and of an ecstatic vision. The most common form of mystical prayer is the prayer of contemplation in which the mystic offers no petition but by gazing upon the Eternal Beauty passes from a state of absorbed attention to an adoration that bursts into rapturous praise. The ecstatic element in such prayer is normally followed by a strong impulse to action. 'The sorrow and the distress which [such] souls felt because they could not die and enjoy our Lord's presence are now exchanged for as fervent a desire for serving Him, of causing Him to be praised, and of helping

[1] Meister Eckhart urged that: 'We ought to pray so fervently that all our organs and powers, both eyes and ears, heart, mouth and all our senses are absorbed in it, and we should not cease till we discover that we desire to be united to Him whom we have present and to whom we pray, that is God.' Quoted: Heiler: op. cit. p. 174.

[2] Cf. this with a passage in the *Bhagavad-Gītā*: 'By giving up self (the ego), force, pride, lust, anger, and acquisitiveness, with no thought of "mine", at peace, so is a man fitted to realize his eternal essence. Become eternal (*brahma-bhūta*), his soul all stilled, he grieves not nor does he desire. Feeling equanimity towards all creatures, he receives the highest love (*bhakti*) of Me. By his loving devotion he comes to *know* Me as I am, how great I am and Who. Then once he has known Me as I am, he forthwith comes to Me.' *Gita*: 18. 53–5: quoted by R. C. Zaehner: *At Sundry Times* (1958) p. 132.

others to the utmost of their power.' [1] It is interesting to note that for mystics in all religions the 'ladder' of prayer includes these processes of recollection, meditation, contemplation, union and ecstasy – processes which are virtually the same for neo-Platonic, Sufi, Hindu and Christian mystics. All are agreed on the use of these approaches to Reality, and all agree that

> in ourselves, we have no power or means to attain to it. . . . Neither mortification, nor purity of heart, nor humility, nor meditation of point after point, nor the most strenuous exercise of affective aspiration, nor all these together, can ever produce a state near enough to contemplation to pass into that perfect state by its own force and weight.[2]

As we said, quoting St Bernard of Clairvaux, the incidence of such prayer is always unexpected, 'I have never at any time been aware of the moment of His coming.' But how, when the mystical moment occurs, can it be described? This brings us to a debatable aspect of mystical language – its erotic character.

Mystical Prayer and Erotic Language

Freud's contention that religion is nothing but a sublimation of the sexual libido seems to receive support from the kind of language most frequently used in certain forms of mystical prayer and experience. On this matter of language, Freud adopts a suggestion by the Swedish philologist, H. Sperber, that sexual needs played a decisive part in the origin and development of language.[3] He argues that language is derived from the mating calls of animals. Language is a sublimated sexuality and, as such, is a crucial instrument in the general deflection of libido from sexual to social ends. This suggestion is discussed by Professor Norman O. Brown who says, in a chapter on 'Language and Eros', that if 'language is made out of (sublimated) sexuality it can hardly be genital sexuality (the mating call of animals)'.[4] Language originates from the development of the child in that general pattern of play, pleasure and love which characterizes the child's relation with his mother. Not until later on does language become the means of communication in the workaday world; such language is an 'operational' superstructure erected upon the erotic basis of child-and-mother relationship.

[1] St Teresa: *The Interior Castle*: 7. iii. 5: Eng. trans. 1912.
[2] Bishop Hedley, quoted by Dom Cuthbert Butler O.S.B.: *Western Mysticism*: Grey Arrow edn (1960) p. 22.
[3] Freud: *Introductory Lectures on Psycho-Analysis* (1940) pp. 140 ff.
[4] Norman O. Brown: *Life Against Death* (1959) pp. 68 ff.

Dr Brown points out that the mystical tradition has long recognized the erotic basis of language. In much the same way as the poet Rainer Maria Rilke (d. 1926) refers to the 'natural speech of the body' so, three centuries earlier, the German mystic, Jacob Boehme, says that Adam's language was an 'unclouded mirror of the senses', being the language spoken by man in paradise. As the result of the Fall,

> No people understands any more the sensual language, but the birds in the air and the beasts in the forest do understand it according to their species. Therefore man may reflect what he has been robbed of, and what he is to recover in the second birth. For in the sensual language all spirits speak with each other, they need no other language, for it is the language of nature.[1]

The pattern of mystical language in the West was established several centuries before Boehme's enunciation of the *sensual* language of paradise. St Bernard's commentary on the *Song of Solomon* may be said to have set the linguistic pattern for 'nuptial' mysticism.

> Neither the pagan nor the Jew, therefore, is so pricked by the darts of love, as is the Church, who says 'I am wounded with love,' and again, 'Stay me with flowers, comfort me with fruits, for I am sick with love.' . . . The fruits the Bride gathers from the Tree of Life when she is brought into the Beloved's garden are pomegranates that take their savour from the Bread of Heaven, their colour from Christ's blood. . . . And yet she [the bride] needs these aids only until such time as all her longings are fulfilled and the Beloved leads her to His chamber, and takes her in His arms and she can say, 'His left hand is under my head, and His right hand doth embrace me. . . .'[2]

This pattern of nuptial symbolism was developed chiefly by Suso and Jacopone da Todi, and exemplified by the devotion of St John of the Cross and St Teresa.

Upon my flowering breast,
His only, as no man but he might prove,
Here slumbering, did he rest,
'Neath my caressing love,
Fann'd by the cedars swaying high above.

When from the turret's height
Scattering his Locks, the breezes play'd around,

[1] Boehme: *Mysterium Magnum*: chap. 35: sec. 59–60.
[2] St Bernard of Clairvaux: *On the Love of God*: newly rendered into English by a Religious of C.S.M.V. (1950) pp. 24–9.

With touch serene and light
He dealt me love's sweet wound,
And with the joyful pain thereof I swoon'd.

Forgetful, rapt, I lay,
My face reclining on my lov'd one fair.
All things for me that day
Ceas'd, as I slumber'd there,
Amid the lilies drowning all my care.[1]

This pattern of Our Lord as the Bridegroom of men's souls (we are reminded that the soul of the male is always described as female – *anima*, that is the 'bride') is not, however, peculiar to medieval Catholicism. It is to be seen in the passionately erotic character of both German and Dutch piety as well as in Sufism and in Hinduism where, for instance, the relationship between Krishna, as an *avatar* of Vishnu, and the human worshipper is expressed in language that is common to the nuptial mysticism of East and West. The use of such language seems to be in the nature of a sublimated sexual activity. It is true that the control of the sexual impulses forms an essential part of the preparation for mystical prayer, and that it is possible that the use of erotic language may be an indirect means of satisfying these deflected sexual impulses, but even so there are other explanations. For instance, the use of erotic language in religion may possibly have its origin in the ancient fertility rites associated with religion in agricultural and pastoral societies. But, perhaps, it is safer to suggest that the desire for, and the sense of, mystical union find their most natural expression in erotic language just because there is no other kind of language sufficiently vivid and sufficiently instinctual to serve as the sublimated expression of man's sense of union with the Beloved.

The word 'love' in a mystical context implies a belief in the existence of a metaphysical reality with which it is 'natural' for the soul to seek union. In the same way as the sexual instinct implies the existence of a human partner with whom physical satisfaction is possible, so mystical impulses imply the existence of a divine Lover, and if this is so, the language of erotic union is natural in such contexts. 'There is

[1] Stanzas from *Spiritual Canticle – Songs between the Soul and the Spouse*: trans. from the Spanish by E. Allison Peers: *Songs of the Lover and the Beloved* (1931) pp. 20 ff.

no space between the Soul and the Highest Good; they are no longer two, but both are united in one; they cannot be separated from each other so long as one is there. This union is imitated in this world by lovers and loved when they wish to unite in one being.'[1]

Mystical and Prophetical Religions

A distinction drawn by Archbishop Söderblom between two types of religion, those which are personality-affirming and those which are personality-denying, is akin to a classification which applies to all the great religions of the world. Some religions, such as Hinduism and Buddhism, are known as 'mystical' religions, while Judaism, Zoroastrianism, Muhammadanism and, in certain of its aspects, Christianity, are called 'prophetical' religions. The adherents of mystical religions feel compelled to empty their psychical life (Suso's 'ceasing to be a creature') in order to achieve by personality-denying techniques an 'emptiness' that will prepare the way for the incoming of the divine. Prophetical religions are personality-affirming, seeking for an active co-operation between the self and the divine. Faith and trust are the key-words of prophetical religions, nuptial love and divine union are the pass-words in mystical religions. One believes in life, the other treats it as an illusion (*maya*), as something to be avoided and finally suppressed. Psychologically, mystical religions represent the feminine side of human nature; the soul plays the woman's part in the nuptial converse with God.

As a result of these differences, each has its own attitude to prayer. Mystical prayer is the prayer of communion and has its own techniques of meditation, contemplation and the suppression of the self. The prayers of prophetical religions emphasize the individual's own existence, his longing for grace and need of personal salvation; it is a more or less spontaneous petition (proceeding from the unconscious) expressing, often vehemently, a sense of profound and exhausting need. It is the type of prayer that proceeds from a guilt-laden soul pleading fearfully for redemption. Yet both forms of prayers, mystical and prophetical, are expressive of a deep spiritual yearning whether such a yearning shows itself as proceeding from a personality-affirming or personality-denying attitude. Whether it accepts the world or rejects it, man's soul seeks for union with another Self. The words of Isaac Pennington (1616–1679) when visiting a Friends' Meeting for the first time express that sense of deep satis-

[1] *Plotinus*: quoted by Heiler: op. cit. p. 214.

faction which is the desire of men in all kinds of religion, and the end for which prayers of all kinds are uttered:

> The presence and power of the Most High reached my heart and conscience. I did not only feel words and demonstrations from without, I felt the dead quickened and the seed raised up, in so much that my heart said: 'This is He, there is no other! This is He whom I have waited for and sought after from my childhood. . . .' [1]

Every mystical religion has its prophetical aspect, and every prophetical religion has its mystical counterpart; the personality-denying and the personality-affirming each prays in its own way, but all seek some Object, State or Person in whom the divisions of this world are resolved.

* * *

Addendum: Children and Prayer

This short section, which belongs to 'The Growth of Religious Consciousness', is added here because it follows more naturally after a discussion of prayer as an adult activity.

For the young child praying is part of a general behaviour pattern, though this pattern appears to be less general today than it once was. Prayer first becomes familiar to the child at its mother's knee, but after a while the child learns that what seemed to be a conversation with a parent is really a conversation directed to some other self than the father or mother.[2] The effect of this instruction sometimes continues into adult life, so that some adults continue to pray in a manner that reflects a childlike rather than an adult attitude to life. Others pray because their experience as children seems to have strengthened the tendencies of the human psyche to express its needs in a real 'conversation' with the divine.

The child after a time discovers intellectual differences between the teaching given by his parents and the world of external circumstances. An eight-year-old child who had been taught that 'faith will move mountains', went on a visit to the White Mountains and prayed for three hours that Mount Washington might be cast into the sea. The negative result so disturbed the child's faith that she could not be induced to pray again for several months.[3] Some children grow to

[1] Isaac Pennington: quoted by Rufus Jones: op. cit. p. 128.

[2] See L. W. Grensted: *The Psychology of Religion* (1952) pp. 126 ff.

[3] See J. B. Pratt: op. cit. pp. 101 ff.

adolescence without experiencing such difficulties, but for many children a critical attitude develops before adolescence. Edmund Gosse tells how as a young child his parents had told him that

> whatever you need, tell Him and He will grant it, if it is His will. Very well: I had need of a large painted humming-top which I had seen in the shop window in the Caledonian Road. Accordingly, I introduced a supplication for this object into my evening prayer, carefully adding the words, 'If it is Thy will.' . . . my Father told me that I must not pray for 'things like that'. To which I answered . . . that I needed the humming-top a great deal more than I did the conversion of the heathen or the restitution of Jerusalem to the Jews, two objects of my nightly supplication which left me very cold.[1]

The intellectual difficulties of petitionary prayer in childhood often persist into adult life and these continue chiefly because the adult individual does not realize that he himself plays an essential part in the 'answer' (whatever it may be) to his intercession. 'Just as we require a point of contact to move the bar of a lever, so God wills that all the action of Heaven on earth should have a point of contact here on earth.' [2] How such a point of contact is established is not a matter we can discuss here, but it should be noted that it involves a realization by the individual that he does not exist *in vacuo*. The individual must come to a lively appreciation of the solidarity of the human race, or, to put it into psychological terms, he must be aware of the extent to which his conscious life is rooted in the pyschical life of mankind. A man at prayer should realize that because of this psychical 'community' he himself may become the medium whereby the prayers of others may be answered. This is a lesson which the young in their intellectual difficulties cannot be expected to understand because the child, as a child, thinks of himself as the natural centre of his own somewhat restricted universe.[3]

[1] Edmund Gosse: *Father and Son*: Evergreen Books edn, p. 41.

[2] See Jacques Maritain: *Degrees of Knowledge* (1937) p. 449, quoted H. Northcott: *The Venture of Prayer* (1951) p. 137.

[3] See J. W. D. Smith: *Psychology and Religion in Early Childhood* (revised edn 1953).

Chapter X

THE PSYCHOLOGY OF RELIGIOUS PRACTICES – WORSHIP

Although worship and prayer are intimately related activities of the soul, the sense of the numinous is more obvious in worship than it generally is in prayer. In worship, adoration replaces intercession, praise, petition. Man from the beginning of his planetary experience has had feelings of an indefinable Something which, whether it be associated with *mana* or some form of animism, totemism or nature, have found their communal expression in ritual patterns which, once established, admit of little variation. The communal nature of worship arose from the fact that the life of primitive man was so closely identified with the life of the group that his conscious activities were dominated by the collective psyche. 'Religious acts are themselves an organic part of the activities of the social body. They are, in fact, social acts.' [1] But it must be noted that these social acts are of a particular kind since they involve, as other social activities do not, a peculiarly vivid appreciation of the Sacred.

The Nature of Worship

Worship is the expression, whether spontaneous or formal, of what man feels and does when in the presence of the Holy. The prostrate body, the clasped hands, the awestruck silence, the cold perspiration, the trembling sense of wonder and fear, are all part of that expression of humility which McDougall called 'self-abasement'. Since man's response to the numinous is something that cannot be fully expressed in rational terms, man has in his worship to employ those symbols which are the precipitate of religious experience down the ages. These symbols appear in a wide variety of religions because they are expressive of psychical elements which are common to all forms of worship, to primitive no less than to the highly liturgical.

[1] Irving King: *The Development of Religion* (1910) p. 122.

An arresting description of a typical act of Hindu worship offers an excellent example of the psychological elements operative in communal forms of worship.

> The drums are beating violently, as he approaches, and the wild music of strange sorts is issuing from the equally strange buildings. . . . On the walls of the rooms are hideous images, carved in stone and daubed with red paint, one representing a monkey, one a creature with a fat human belly and an elephant's head; each with an offering of yellow marigolds before it; while in the most prominent place is a stone pillar, rounded off on the top, wet from the pouring of much Ganges water, bedaubed with spots of paint and surrounded with green leaves, uncooked rice, a few coins, and more yellow marigolds. There are two priests in the corner, beating tom-toms, and by the pillar stands a third, daubing it with more paint, pouring water over it, placing leaves upon it, and all the while mumbling words – many of them mere repetitions of names – to which no one seems to listen. The noise becomes louder, and the old priest seizes a lighted lamp and brandishes it about in front of the much-bedaubed pillar, while the audience follow his motions with obvious excitement; and at the close of the hocus-pocus he distributes to them some of the rice which he has collected at the foot of the sacred object.[1] The performance has been unintelligible to our visitor, but the most astonishing thing about it all is the attitude and aspect of the worshippers. For worshippers they indubitably are. Some of them have been standing, some kneeling, some prostrate on their faces. Each has made an offering before the bedrenched pillar or at the feet of the bedrenched figures on the walls, and though some seem indifferent, many give unmistakable signs of reverence, that they have found in that preposterous transaction the same sort of inner treasure which our Protestant churchgoer has occasionally carried home with him on a Sunday from his American meeting-house.[2]

The visitor is reported as asking 'Why do they go through these absurd actions? How did the thing ever start and why do they keep it

[1] Linga (phallus) worship plays a prominent part in all the religions of India where the lingam is the symbol of Siva, occupying the central position in large shrines found in all parts of the sub-continent. Phallic cults associated with stones of significant shapes, large pillars and trees are to be found in Greek and Semitic religions, while processions carrying phallic symbols play as prominent a part in the Holī celebrations of India as they did formerly in the Dionysian rites of the classical world. In fertility rites, Vishnu is represented as fertilizing the earth by scattering phallic fragments all over the world, the same ritual intention as figured in the distribution of mutilated fragments of the body of Osiris. Such acts are symbolical representations of man's veneration of the gods or principles responsible for reproduction, birth and new life. It is not surprising, therefore, that Freud should view such practices as supporting his contention that religion and culture are nothing but elaborations of the sexual instinct.

[2] J. B. Pratt: *The Religious Consciousness* (1930) pp. 255–6.

up?' But what are here called 'absurd actions' have their counterpart in the religions of the West, whether it be in a weekly assembly which listens intently to one of its members reading from a laige sacred book passages which have strong numinous associations, after which those present stand to sing and subsequently place coins in a collecting bag; or, another assembly which with elaborate ceremonial shares a common token meal which is said to be the Sacred Body and Blood of the Adored Being. Despite their outward and visible differences, religious cults, both East and West, in their worship – whatever their theology – have a common psychological basis.

It is important to emphasize the commonness of these psychological motivations, because the various forms of worship are sometimes somewhat arbitrarily classified as 'objective' and 'subjective'. Objective worship is described as that which aims to make some effect upon the deity worshipped; subjective worship is that which aims to make some impression upon the worshipper. But the plain fact is that even if the worshipper's intention is to concentrate upon the Object to which worship is directed, every worshipful act has its subjective effect upon those participating in that worship. Hindu worship is said to be objective since its temples and its services are designed for the benefit and honour of the gods rather than for the benefit of the worshipper. But this statement needs qualifying if we consider the obvious subjective effects which Hindu worship has upon its participants. On the other hand, Jainism (whose gods are sunk in an eternal sleep) and Buddhism are described as being subjective in their forms of worship. None the less Buddhism, despite its original non-theistic attitude, in the course of time assimilated many of the 'objective' practices of Hindu worship, so that the relationship of the subjective and objective elements in Buddhist worship is particularly close.[1] The later books of the *Upanishads* make it clear that Hinduism recognized a trinity of elements in its worship, (*a*) the multitudinous members of the Hindu pantheon who were manifestations of the godhead, Brahmā, (*b*) the *impulse* to worship, and (*c*) the worshipper himself. Since these three elements are active in all forms of worship, it is questionable whether it is psychologically correct to make too sharp a distinction between objective and subjective aspects of

[1] Mahāyāna Buddhism (the Greater Vehicle) has elevated the historical Buddha, who dismissed all discussions about the existence of deities, into a theistic Image so that he and his manifestations (the Boddhisatvas) have become the object of devoutly reverent worship.

worship. The one inevitably implies (even if it does not assert) the existence of the other.

When we turn to Christian forms of worship it is sometimes argued that Catholic worship, with its vestments, ornaments and furnishings of sanctuary, altar and shrines, is objectively directed to the glory of God, while Protestant worship, both in its forms and settings, is designed primarily for the sake of the congregation, or, as Pratt says, 'for the audience'.[1] But Pratt had to admit that even the most objective forms of worship affect the worshipper who may find that 'a church in which mass is being said is an excellent place to pray, that the service gives him an intense realisation of the closeness of God to human life, and that he goes away from it with a sense of spiritual refreshment'.[2] Architecture, decoration, ornaments, hymns, music, ritual and the sermon (which plays a more prominent part in Protestant than in Catholic worship) exercise collectively and separately an effect upon the congregation, strengthening their faith and elevating their moral and spiritual outlook. Every form of worship and every act of prayer is at one and the same time embracive of the worshipper and the supernatural. The educated critical 'observer', no less than the most naïve believer, may sometimes feel in a worshipful setting the same sense of the High and the Holy.

Rebecca West, in an eloquent and highly descriptive passage, relates how as a visitor she was present in the Patriarchate Church in Frushka Gora (in what was then Serbia) accompanied by a guide who was a non-believer and who felt obliged to apologize for having taken his visitor to the church during the course of a service.

> In the white and gold theatre of a baroque church the students of the theological seminary attached to the Patriarchate were assisting at a Lenten mass. The priests passed in and out of the royal door in the great iconostasis, which framed in gilt the richness of the holy pictures. As they came and went there could be seen for an instant the shining glory of the altar, so sacred that it must be hidden lest the people look at it so long that they forget its nature, as those who stare at the sun see in time not the source of light but the black circle. The students' voices

---

[1] It is difficult to maintain this distinction in Anglican worship. The Prayer Book of 1549 explains that a Common Book was issued in the common tongue, and its orders, ceremonies and readings are designed 'so that every man may understand what they do mean and what use they do serve'. This intention of making worship intelligible to the congregation was accompanied by a corresponding intention 'to please God' – a liturgical balance between the subjective and the objective.

[2] Pratt: op. cit. p. 299.

> affirmed the glory of the hidden altar, and declared what it was that makes it adorable, what loveliness is and harmony. The unfolding of the rite brought us all down on our knees in true prostration, with the forehead bent to the floor. 'It is only necessary to do this during Holy Week,' gasped Constantine apologetically in my ear. 'I am so very sorry.' He thought that English dignity would be affronted by the necessity to adopt this attitude. But there could have been nothing more agreeable than to be given the opportunity to join in this ceremony which, if nothing in the Christian legend were true, would still be uplifting and fortifying, since it proclaims that certain elements in experience are supremely beautiful and that we should grudge them nothing of our love and service. It inoculated man against his constant and disgusting madness, his preference for the disagreeable over the agreeable. Here was the unique accomplishment of the Eastern Church. It was the child of Byzantium, a civilization which had preferred the visual arts to literature, and had been divided from the intellectualized West by a widening gulf for fifteen hundred years. . . . It devoted all its forces to the achievement of the mass, the communal form of art which might enable man from time to time to apprehend why it is believed that there may be a God.[1]

This lively account of the effect of a 'foreign' form of worship upon a non-believer, brings to our attention the part played by the aesthetic element in religion, and particularly in worship.

Aesthetics and Worship

The effect that so-called objective forms of worship have upon the worshipper is particularly clear when we consider the part played by the aesthetic elements in corporate acts of worship.

In many religions, Christian and non-Christian alike, the sense of the Objective Presence is stimulated by tangible and visible aids to worship. This is as true for primitive man as it is for the religions of highly civilized societies, hence the psychological efficacy of fetiches, the use of the *churinga* among Australian Aruntas, *yantras* among Hindu yogin, *mandalas* among Buddhist contemplatives, crucifixes, rosaries, burning lamps, images of the Virgin and Child, tabernacles containing the Blessed Sacrament, shrines furnished with such sacred relics as the bone of a saint, a tooth of the Buddha, or a fragment of the True Cross. The subjective attitude of those to whom such objects are of value varies according to the intellectual and cultural level of the worshipper, but the use of sacred objects as aids to concentration in worship and meditation is everywhere an eloquent witness to the subjective element in worship. For instance, we find St John of the Cross in the *Ascent of Mount Carmel* saying that 'creatures' help to

[1] Rebecca West: *Black Lamb and Grey Falcon*: Vol. I. pp. 518 ff. (1955).

serve as a revelation of God, and he suggests a test by which our sensory experiences may be judged to be spiritually profitable:

> It is that, whensoever a person hears music and other things, and sees pleasant things, and is conscious of sweet perfumes, or tastes things that are delicious, or feels soft touches, if his thought and the affection of his will are at once centred upon God and if that thought of God gives him more pleasure than the movement of the sense which causes it, and save for that he finds no pleasure in the said movement, that is a sign that he is receiving benefit therefrom, and that this thing of sense is a help to his spirit. In this way such things may be used, for then such things of sense subserve the end for which He created and gave them, which is that He should be the better loved and known because of them.[1]

Such objects are not only focal points for worshipful concentration, their associated 'sacredness' when presented aesthetically (even if crudely) reinforces the worshipper's apprehension of the Holy.

It is true that the use or creation of aesthetic adjuncts to worship is not always based on purely religious motives. Many great buildings are said to have been designed and adorned in honour of deity, but the motives behind such erections are sometimes rather mixed. The size or design of a temple, ziggurat, cathedral or church spire may be dictated by a certain competitive ambition which prompts a city or a community to surpass its commercial or political rivals. Many of the great churches of East Anglia show quite clearly that their aesthetic excellence is in some measure indebted to the competitive ambitions of their founders, the medieval wool-merchants. But the psychological elements in religious aestheticism are basically the same for all religions. This statement receives support from an argument persuasively presented by Dean Dillistone:

> Are not man's symbolic activities of two kinds? On the one hand he desires to ascend *upwards*. He wishes to grow. . . . He desires to lift his dependents, his possessions, his powers to higher levels of existence, than they at present occupy. So in his ritual activities, he *raises, lifts, offers*. But concurrently he *repudiates, renounces, annuls*. He separates himself from the low and the downward-dragging in order that he may rise to the high and upward-rising. In his architecture, in his art, in his ritual activities, this is the pattern we find expressed again and again. In his upward spirit man cries:
>
> 'Lift every gift that Thou Thyself hast given,
> Low lies the best till lifted up to heav'n.'[2]

---

[1] St John of the Cross: *Ascent of Mount Carmel*: III. xxiv (Works. I. 284), quoted by E. Allison Peers: *Spirit of Flame* (1947) pp. 147–8.

[2] F. W. Dillistone: *Christianity and Symbolism* (1955) pp. 261–2.

But, in addition to this upward-directed activity,[1]

> man desires to move *forward.* He wishes to advance. He yearns for a better country, for a better order of society. He feels the pull towards the future. He craves the companionship of others in this common quest. He dies to the past in order that he may live to the future.[2]

These two impulses, the upward-moving and the forward-seeking, are two of the most powerful subjective elements in religion and religious art.[3] The upward-seeking impulse explains the heavenward pointing towers, spires and arches of Gothic Christendom, the lofty platforms, rising tier upon tier as in the Boro-Budur, in Babylonian ziggurats and the pyramidal temples of ancient Mexico and the design of Tibetan *stupas.*[4] It explains the age-old habit of building shrines and churches upon high hills, even as Semitic peoples erected altars on 'high places'. It explains the belief that the gods lived in successive stages of the heavenly places, rising to a final 'floor' where dwelt the Supreme Deity.

[1] This has been the subject of comment both by von Hügel and W. R. Inge. The former held that 'the satisfaction of man's natural impulses and instincts on a normal level is not enough to content him, and the more refined and sensitive his nature, the greater is his discontent. There is what is called in modern language an "urge" upwards.' L. V. Lester-Garland: *The Religious Philosophy of Baron F. von Hügel* (1933) p. 75. Inge frequently quoted Plotinus who 'would have us believe that all things are naturally attracted upwards to the sphere next above them: as Proclus puts it in a striking phrase, "all things pray, except the Supreme".' W. R. Inge: *Vale* (1934) p. 52.

[2] op. cit. p. 262.

[3] The upward thrusting impulse in religious architecture has also a psychoanalytical explanation. Jung describes a dream he had as a boy aged four which made a permanent impression upon him, but it was not until quite late in life that he realized the psychological significance of what he had seen on a red cushion resting on a large golden throne in a deep rectangular stone basement. This had a tree trunk about twelve inches high with a sort of fleshy head that was not like a head but had an opening like the eye of a demon. What he had seen was a phallic archetype, 'the principle of creativity which is expressed in many forms, such as the resurrection of life, the minaret, the pillar-like grave monuments in Turkey, Assam and elsewhere, the towers on churches and so on'. Quoted by E. A. Bennet: *C. G. Jung* (1961) pp. 10 ff. To which we may add that the uprising features of religious architecture may be interpreted as the sublimated objectification of an impulse which, whether it be described analytically as a sexual archetype, philosophically as man's search for some *telos* or as a religious aspiration for the Divine, is an impulse whose purpose is to lift man's spirit to the higher levels of existence.

[4] Tibetan and Chinese *stupas* are impressive architectural combinations of certain fundamental shapes, a square or cube, surmounted by a circle or sphere, surmounted by a triangle or pyramid, a pillar and a crescent, shapes which are spiritually significant in all religions. See Paul Carus: *Chinese Thought* (1907) for several illustrations and a full explanation of these architectural symbolisms.

The forward-moving impulse finds its architectural expression in the long avenues of megalithic monuments, in the processional routes of Egyptian temples and classical religions, in the long naves and ambulatories of Gothic buildings culminating in the High Altar. Furthermore, these two impulses together furnish a psychological explanation of the fact that many religions in their architectural settings have impressive ceremonial stairways (quite independent of the nature of the actual site) whether they be the long processional inclines of a Babylonian ziggurat, the various versions of the *Via Sacra* or the steps cut in the pillar or tree which in Shamanism connects earth and heaven (cf. Jacob's dream of the *ladder*).

A third impulse explains the circularity which distinguishes so much of the world's religious architecture and ritual. The circular tumuli, the stone circles of megalithic art, the concentric circles of primitive rock scribblings, the circular designs of mosaic pavements in French, Italian and Spanish churches, the legendary Labyrinth of Crete, no less than Botticelli's illustrations of the *Candida Rosa* of Dante's *Paradiso,* and the domes which surmount so many of the world's temples and churches, all are the aesthetic expression of man's desire to return to that centre from which he himself first came. This regressive tendency is seen in the mythology of the *Omphalos* – the Navel of the Earth. This particular myth, as Professor Mircea Eliade has pointed out, has its architectural expressions in the religions of Vedic India, China, in Teutonic mythology and also in Christianity. Such visible expressions of this impulse may be interpreted in terms of the Freudian Oedipus Complex, in terms of man's desire to return to the Mother. The Omphalos is the symbolic expression of the belief that 'The Holy One created the world like an embryo. As the embryo proceeds from the navel outwards, so God began to create the world from its navel outwards and from there it was spread out in different directions.' [1] Rudolf Otto allied these various psychological motivations with man's sense of the numinous, explaining that it is this combination which is responsible for some of the magnificent forms of religious art.

> In the arts nearly everywhere the most effective means of representing the numinous is the 'sublime'. This is especially true of architecture, in which it would appear to have first been realized. One can hardly escape

[1] A. J. Wensinck: *The Idea of the Western Semites concerning the Navel of the Earth*: Amsterdam (1926).

the idea that this feeling for expression must have begun to awaken far back in the remote Megalithic age.[1]

The architecture which in the West most movingly expresses these psychological impulses and this feeling of the numinous, is without doubt to be found in Byzantine churches which, by combining the shapes of the Circle, the Square and the Cross,[2] achieve an architectural symbolism which is a visible fusion of Christian belief and the sense of the numinous.

> Let us enter into a cross-in-square church and strive to apprehend its spirit. It is of moderate, perhaps even of modest, dimensions, and the wide extent of unbroken floor space is much diminished. Yet the majestic and transcendental spirit and the sense of spaciousness and freedom are indubitably present. The presence of the Infinite and eternal God is still expressed. If we stand beneath the dome and look upwards we realize it. . . . It is the dome which chiefly contributes to the sense of the infinite and the sublime. It lifts itself above us, illuminated by the windows which surround it, and as the gaze rests within it, the mind feels the sense of the majestic and the sublime. Moreover, by the insertion of the cylindrical drum, the portrait of Christ the Almighty is thrust into a remoter distance. Dwelling in light inaccessible, He looks down from His lofty height and the sides of the drum are utilized to furnish Him with the guard of bejewelled angels to signalize His glory.[3]

Byzantine architecture is not only the most balanced expression of the subjective and objective elements in religion it is also a superb embodiment of the fundamental motives operative in religious practice.[4]

[1] Rudolf Otto: *The Idea of the Holy* (1950) p. 68.

[2] In a succinct article on the symbolism of Architecture, Señor J. E. Cirlot points to an interesting connexion between the squaring of the circle in Buddhist *mandalas* and *stupas* and the symbolism of the dome, circle, square and cross in Romanesque churches. See J. E. Cirlot: *A Dictionary of Symbols* (trans. from the Spanish by Jack Sage) (1962) pp. 15 ff.

[3] J. Arnott Hamilton: *Byzantine Architecture and Decoration* (1956) pp. 276 ff. This work has an impressive set of illustrations.

[4] An arresting account of the effect of worship within a setting of great architectural splendour relates to the visit paid by 'ten wise men from Kiev' to Constantinople, at the end of the tenth century. The delegation had been sent by Prince Vladimir to investigate on its own ground the new religion (Christianity) that was being offered to the Russians by the Eastern Orthodox Church. 'As the light from thousands of candles gleamed on the polished surface of green marble and purple porphyry [in Santa Sophia], as the figures of austere saints and bejewelled emperors looked down from the encrusted walls, as the wings of the seraphs lay outstretched in the pendentives far above, as the clouds of incense floated through the expanse, as the priests in their silken vestments moved slowly in procession, as the celebrant passed through the iconostasis into the presence of the altar, as a great multitude stood in rapt devotion and as the solemn chant echoed through the nave, it is no wonder that the visitors from the Russian plains

The Worshipper Participates

We now have to turn to the more personal aspects of worship. The emotional effects of public worship are greatly intensified if the worshipper himself is able to participate physically in the actual rite – quite independent of whether it be a simple or an elaborate form of worship.

It is a well-known fact that kinaesthetic sensations play an essential part in many emotional experiences; it is important to note that they often play a similar rôle in acts of worship. If the worshipper plays an instrument, carries a banner, holds a lighted candle, or walks in a procession, his emotional response is considerably increased by such physical participation. If the worshipper participates by joining in responses or by singing, particularly if the setting is both rhythmical and uplifting, his respiration and circulation will be correspondingly affected.

In most religions, kinaesthetic sensations are associated with forms of worship whose ritual acts, resonant tones, colourful presentation, olfactory stimuli, historical associations and reverential gestures create an atmosphere of great solemnity. The pouring of water over a *lingam* no less than signing oneself with holy water can evoke a more satisfying emotional response than if the intending worshipper is merely a passive spectator. Genuflexions, prostrations, the kissing of some sacred relic, the offering of a sacramental gift, all such actions intensify not only the worshipper's emotions but also the vitality of his worship,[1] provided that such ritual activities are not alien to his temperament or inherited tradition.

---

felt the throb of an unprecedented emotion in their souls, and beheld mingling with the worshippers angelic visitants from heaven.' J. Arnott Hamilton: op. cit. p. 79. See also Nicolas Zernov: *The Russian Prophets* (1944) p. 18, who commenting on this historical visit says: 'The beauty and splendour of that worship was so magnificent that the Russian envoys did not know whether they were still on earth or already in heaven.' As a result of this visit, Prince Vladimir and his Council joined the Eastern Orthodox Church, and Christianity was brought into Russia.

[1] The connexion between religion and physical movement is emphasized by Sir Maurice Bowra in his brilliant study of *Primitive Song* in which he says that among primitive peoples 'singing is often accompanied by some kind of action, such as a dance, in which bodily movements are repeated on various patterns, or mimetic gestures, which illustrate what the words say and make their references and implications more forceful'. He suggests that primitive song had its origin in rhythmical physical gestures which enable a community to express profound

Worship – Sound and Silence

The part played by sound and silence in worship is of vital importance. It is significant that although the language used in some religious rites may be incomprehensible to the worshipper, it is psychologically effective if it carries with it overtones of a numinous character. The sound of distant solemn music, or of singing heard behind choir screens in cathedral or monastic churches, promotes a general worshipful feeling. Even in forms designed to make the course of public worship intelligible to those present, a worshipful atmosphere is achieved by the familiar cadences of biblical readings, psalms and public prayers (whether liturgical or extemporaneous) with their traditional invocations and terminal phraseology, all of which help to create a certain numinosity.[1]

A modern example of the effect of words solemnly uttered in the presence of a congregation is to be found in the experience of a young intelligent agnostic who, having no previous knowledge of Christian worship, was taken to evensong in a parish church for the first time on Palm Sunday.

> My first experience of the worship of the Church was evensong on Palm Sunday. As it was my first visit to a church most of my time was spent looking round and about, and the thing that struck me, especially during the prayers, was the rapt attention of all present on what they were doing; all heads were bowed, and at the end of each prayer the whole body of people seemed to say Amen as one man. . . . I really felt that those

---

emotions when confronted with the supernatural. C. M. Bowra: *Primitive Song* (1962) pp. 28–33.

Among these rhythmical gestures, dancing is one of the most important means of communal expression. 'The dance is one of man's earliest attempts to move in an imaginary world of his own creation, which none the less stands in a close relation to the actual world and fulfils some function in it whether magical or religious or ceremonial or merely diverting. . . . Through dances primitive peoples express their emotions with all the force that dancing allows, and work an enchantment on some prey or show their identity with their totems or illustrate some myth or hold intercourse with their gods. All these things their songs also do, but without the dance, the song would hardly exist . . .' (op. cit. pp. 261–2).

[1] Le Bon, dealing with the effect of words on the masses, observed that: 'Words handled with art . . . possess in sober truth the mysterious power formerly attributed to them by the adepts of magic. They cause the birth in the minds of the crowd of the most formidable tempest, which in turn they are capable of stilling. . . . The power of words is bound up with the images they evoke, and is quite independent of their real significance. They are uttered with solemnity in the presence of crowds, and as soon as they have been pronounced, an expression of respect is visible on every countenance and all heads are bowed.' Le Bon: *The Crowd* (1920) pp. 116–18.

people had quite definitely got something that I knew nothing about. . . . There was an atmosphere.[1]

When we turn to consider words that are sung, we find that hymns (particularly those in Christian worship) fall more or less into two categories – those which are intended to uplift or instruct the worshippers, and those which being directed to the Deity carry strong overtones of mystery.[2] One of the most typical of all such hymns is the Trisagion of Bishop Reginald Heber (d. 1826), 'Holy, Holy, Holy, Lord God Almighty!' in which the repetition of the word 'Holy' reinforces the solemnity of this act of vocal praise. Such hymns illustrate the fact that musical sounds heard in a religious context often have the power to affect deeply even those who have repudiated all organized forms of religion. The effect of listening to Plainsong, the Bach *B Minor Mass* or the excitement of Stanford's setting in C of the *Magnificat*[3] can convert (if only temporarily) listeners into worshippers, even if intellectual difficulties had long before caused them to sever their connexions with religion. Such results are in large measure derived from the fact that states of intellectual tension often find a natural relaxation in sounds which are splendidly moving in their composition.

Our understanding of the psychological nature of music used in worship is in a large measure dependent upon our ability to answer the question, 'How did man become musically conscious?' It has been suggested that in so far as music is rhythmical, it may possibly have developed as the result of the sound of rhythmical blows of stone hammers or early metal tools. But it might equally have developed as the result of primitive man's listening to the waves of the sea and the songs of birds. A writer on the folk-music of Norwegian Lapland refers to the fact that people, thought to be descendants of the Lappish Stone Age culture, had folk-songs which are 'songs without words'. A modern Norwegian hearing one of these wordless songs identified the sounds with those of the Arctic *havella* bird, adding that the Lapps believed that such songs had been composed by the

[1] Bryan Green: *The Practice of Evangelism* (1951) p. 62.

[2] Thousands of the hymns written by the Wesleys were designed to stir the emotions of those to whom their sermons were so powerfully addressed. The flamboyant tunes to which many of these hymns were set matched the emotional fervour of those listening to John Wesley preaching out of doors, many of whom fell to the ground, foaming at the mouth.

[3] 'The *Service in C* captures a kind of spacious beauty highly charged emotionally, seraphic at times, and always restrained, which makes it perhaps the best of all his services.' See C. Henry Phillips: *The Singing Church* (1945) p. 225.

birds themselves.[1] It is, however, much more likely that wordless songs originated naturally as vocal expressions of man's emotional reaction to situations of happiness and joy. This agrees with Ralph Vaughan Williams's view that the wordless songs of primitive people are spontaneous expressions of mystical emotions which are beyond words.[2] Such wordless songs (*melismata*) appear as mystical jubilations in Christian liturgical forms.[3]

St Augustine, in his commentary on the Psalms, asks what does singing a Jubilation mean?

> It is the realization that words cannot express the inner music of the heart. For those who sing in the harvest field or vineyard, or in work deeply occupying the attention, when they are overcome with joy at the words of the song, being filled with such exultation, the words fail to express their emotion, so leaving the syllables of the words, they drop into vowel sounds – the vowel sounds signifying that the heart is yearning to express what the tongue cannot utter.[4]

In his commentary on Psalm 100, *Jubilate Deo*, Augustine writes: 'You know already what it is to sing a jubilation, rejoice and speak. If you cannot express your joy, let the jubilation do it, what is more expressive of joy than the jubilation? If speech is not expressive, joy need not therefore be silent.' [5] If Augustine believed that the simple peasant sang with his whole soul from pure joy, then we may accept Rudolph Steiner's views that if we pronounce a *vowel* sound we are giving expression to something that comes from the inmost depths of our being.[6] Jubilation occurs not only in worship, it is also an element in mystical prayer. Richard Rolle of Hampole (d. 1349) says that the man who has given himself by constant devotion to God, receives 'a holy sound from Heaven' which changes thought and

[1] Ragnwald Graff: 'The Music of Norwegian Lapland': *The Journal of the International Folk Music Council*: Vol VI (1954). This resembles Sperber's suggestion that language itself is derived from the mating calls of animals; see p. 125 *supra*.

[2] See Preface to G. B. Chambers: *Folksong – Plainsong* (1956).

[3] See Egon Wellesz: *A History of Byzantine Music and Hymnography* (1949) for a detailed and scholarly account of the origins of early musical forms of Christian worship. St Paul's advice to the early Christians that they should speak to one another (alternatively, 'to yourselves') 'in psalms and hymns and spiritual songs' (Eph. v. 19) is explained by Dr Wellesz who argues that a spiritual song (*ode pneumatike*) is a special kind of jubilation. Such melismatic songs include *Alleluias* and other musical expressions of joy which Jewish Christians brought with them into Christian worship from that of the Temple and the synagogue.

[4] Augustine: commentary on Psalm 32: *Beati quorum remissae sunt iniquitates*: quoted in G. B. Chambers: op. cit. p. 4.

[5] *ibid.* [6] Rudolph Steiner: *Eurhythmy as Visible Speech* (1920) p. 12.

meditation into song. Chambers explains this mystical form of jubilation as a state of ecstasy which proceeds, as does the spontaneous art of the peasant folk-singer, from the depths of man's unconscious nature.[1]

Such studies in folklore provide one more means whereby we may understand the spiritual experiences of our ancient ancestry. Early man's reactions to his environment caused him, in moments of joy, to break into wordless songs,[2] so that these melismatic expressions came naturally to occupy a place in all forms of worship, liturgical and otherwise. Indeed the subjective effectiveness of the Divine Office is in some measure due to the inclusion of such melismatic sounds, since these naturally musical expressions of thankfulness are among the most satisfying elements of worship.[3]

[1] Chambers: op. cit. p. 29.

[2] Discussing the *technique* of Primitive Song, Sir Maurice Bowra says that according to modern notions 'a song consists of words sung by the human voice, but we have no right to assume that the first sounds used in songs were necessarily words in the strict sense of intelligible units of communication. Indeed it is unlikely that they were. Song begins with some sort of tune, and to adapt real words to it is a separate and subsequent task which calls for considerable dexterity. A mere tune, if hummed, can still satisfy its performers, who feel that it expresses something quite adequately, and does not demand words to make it more explicit . . .' (op. cit. p. 57).

In support of this view Bowra refers to a visit paid by H.M.S. *Beagle* to Tierra del Fuego in 1838. It was found that the Yamana natives sang tunes to emotive and unintelligible syllables. 'Such meaningless sounds really look as if they were the earliest kind of songs practised by man' (op. cit. p. 59). The importance of this conclusion for our purpose is that many of these wordless songs seem to be directly related to the fact that man's sense of the supernatural provokes him to sing of that mystery which 'is present both in the visible and in the invisible world, in the life of living things and in the powers which lie within and without them' (op. cit. p. 279).

[3] St John Chrysostom observes that 'nothing so fitly lifts up the soul, and influences it in such a manner when exalted, frees it from earth and looses it from the burdens of the flesh . . . as the singing of musical intervals [i.e. *cantus modulationis* = jubilation], divine song well ordered. Our nature is so constantly delighted with songs and melodies that infants at the breast, if they cry and are troubled are soothed in this way; nurses certainly who carry infants in arms, going to and fro often, are singing to them children's ditties and keep them quiet in this way. Moreover, travellers in the middle of the day, making a journey on yoked animals, sing, finding consolation from the tedium of the journey in these songs. . . . Farm workers treading the grapes in the wine-press, gathering the grapes, or training the vines, and doing any other work whatsoever, frequently sing. Sailors, as well, when rowing, do thus. Women also while weaving, and when separating a tangled warp on the beam, sometimes individually, at other times altogether, sing one particular melody. . . . Where there are spiritual songs, thither the grace of the Spirit hastens, which sanctifies the mouth and the soul.' See Peter Wagner: *History of Plain-Chant* (1901).

But sound has its natural counterpart in silence; in certain contexts it is no less expressive than sound. Molinos, the Quietist, regarded silence as the most natural approach to the Ineffable – 'silence of the mouth, silence of the mind, silence of the will'. The prolonged silence that follows the Elevation of the Host at Mass, or the silence of a Quaker meeting, is consistent with that awesome response which man has made from the earliest times to his apprehension of the presence of the Holy. Silence is as expressive a reaction to epiphanies of the Sacred as are fear-full ejaculations[1] or spontaneous expressions of joy. In the Liturgy of St James, we have a poetical expression of silence as a primeval reaction to the numinous:

Let all mortal flesh keep silence, and with fear and trembling stand
Pondering nothing earthly-minded, for with blessings in his hand
Christ our God to earth descendeth our full homage to demand.

But the concluding verse shows that man's awestruck silence reaches a climax at which it bursts into fervent praise: both are natural reactions to the *numen praesens.*

At his feet the six-winged Seraph: Cherubim with sleepless eye:
Veil their faces to the Presence as with ceaseless voice they cry:
Alleluia, Alleluia, Alleluia, Lord most High!

Silence, whether in liturgical or non-liturgical forms of worship, as a sacramental act is capable of a three-fold analysis. (1) The silence of *waiting* in which those present, having excluded earthly preoccupations, wait for the outpouring of the Spirit.[2] (2) The silence of *communion* among those who feel themselves moved to worship the Ineffable without the hindrance or limitation of language. (3) The silence of *adoration*, the silence of those who in the presence of the

[1] It has been suggested that many 'words' associated with religion were originally ejaculations evoked by a sense of fear in the presence of the Sacred. The Buddhist OM from the Sanskrit HUM no less than the name of the Hebrew YAH may originally have been spontaneous verbal reactions to the *mysterium tremendum et fascinans.* See Rudolf Otto: *The Idea of the Holy*: Appendix III: 'Original Numinous Sounds'.

[2] Charles Lamb in his essay, *A Quakers' Meeting*, says: 'Frequently the Meeting is broken up without a word having been spoken. But the mind has been fed. You go away with a sermon not made with hands. . . . You have bathed in silence. O, when the spirit is sore fretted, even tired to sickness of the janglings and nonsense-noises of the world, what a balm and a solace it is to go and seat yourself for a quiet half-hour upon some undisputed corner of a bench, among the gentle Quakers!'

L

Holy feel a sense of *rapport* which needs neither word nor action – 'prostrate before Thy throne to lie, and gaze and gaze on Thee'. But however expressed, there is yet another form of worship besides those of praise and prayer – perhaps the most ancient and the most expressive of all such forms – sacrifice.

Worship and Sacrifice

Contemporary anthropology, despite earlier objections to Robertson Smith's theory of sacrifice and Freud's much-criticized use of it in *Totem and Taboo*, shows that the drama of sacrifice is one of the earliest and most nearly universal of all religious activities. In fact, what is called an 'altar' may be one of the oldest pieces of 'furniture' in the world. So we have to ask what are the psychological motives behind sacrifice?

Men have offered sacrifices for one or more of three reasons: because (1) they believed it to be the means whereby a gift could be offered to deity either as an act of gratitude, adulation, or as an act of propitiation: because (2) it was one of the most effective means whereby men and deity could share a common life; because (3) it was a means whereby the life of the community or of the world could be sustained. This last motive has its most terrible expression in the sacrifices offered by the Aztec priests. Every day a sacrifice of human hearts torn from the bodies of living victims was offered in order to help the sun to rise. The ancient Mexicans believed that the sun itself had been born from blood and sacrifice.

> It is said that the gods gathered in the twilight at Teotihuacán, and one of them, a little leprous god, covered with boils, threw himself into a huge brazier as a sacrifice. He rose from the blazing coals changed into a sun: but this new sun was motionless; it needed blood to move. So the gods immolated themselves, and the sun, drawing life from their death, began its course across the sky. This was the beginning of the cosmic drama in which humanity took on the rôle of the gods. To keep the sun moving in its course, so that the darkness should not overwhelm the world for ever, it was necessary to feed it every day with its food, 'the precious water' (*chalchiuatl*) – that is, with human blood. . . .
>
> Every time that a priest on the top of a pyramid held up the bleeding heart of a man and then placed it in the *quauhxicalli* [the vessel of the Sun] the disaster that perpetually threatened to fall upon the world was postponed once more. Human sacrifice was an alchemy by which life was made out of death.[1]

---

[1] Jacques Soustelle: *Daily Life of the Aztecs* (1961) pp. 96–7.

Commenting upon how much this aspect of Mexican civilization may shock the modern reader, Soustelle adds that

> Human sacrifice among the Mexicans was inspired neither by cruelty nor by hatred. It was their response to . . . the instability of a continually threatened world. Blood was necessary to save this world and the men in it; the victim was no longer an enemy to be killed, but a messenger, arrayed in a dignity that was almost divine, who was sent to the gods.[1]

Young girls, willing victims, representing the goddess Xilone, were beheaded in a dance at the maize harvest; other women, representing the mother-goddess Xipe Totec, were killed by arrows whilst fastened on a sacrificial frame and then flayed to assist the drying of the maize for the winter's food. The distribution and burial in cultivated fields of portions of the bodies of sacrificed victims was a means of sustaining life through death, a practice found in many parts of the world.

Such sacrifices were accompanied in many religions by communal meals[2] in which the body of the victim or some sacramental equivalent not only reinforced the life of the participants but helped to maintain the universe and the life of the community. The 'maintenance-value' of agricultural sacrifices continued to be highly esteemed even by the great riverine civilizations of the ancient West, for civilization itself required reinforcement by means of this life-through-death ritual. Sacrifices in the temple of Marduk were an epitome of tillage of the land. But these life-maintaining rituals included, as we have already seen, other psychological motives. We have already considered Freud's explanation that sacrificial rituals had their origin in the commemoration of a parricidal murder committed by the members of a horde who, having slain their Leader, ate his body and thereafter instituted a communal meal that was both a means of propitiation and of commemoration. This Freudian explanation may seem alien to the Christian understanding of sacrifice as celebrated in the Mass or Eucharist, but it supports the suggestion

[1] op. cit. p. 99.

[2] Jung quotes from Bernardino de Sahagun, *General History of the Things of New Spain*, who began his missionary work among the Aztecs in 1529, eight years after the conquest of Mexico. He describes how out of a doughlike paste made from the crushed and pounded seeds of the prickly poppy, a figure of the god Huitzilopochtli was moulded. Then the 'god' was slain with a dart, and the body of the god was broken up and distributed in very small fragments. The response of those who had shared this broken sacrificial body was 'The god is eaten'. And those who ate it were described as 'guardians' of the god. See Jung: *Psychology and Religion: West and East*: Vol. 11. pp. 223–4.

that man has offered sacrifices from very early times from a variety of impulses. Prominent among these is the fact that sacrifice always involves a symbolical offering of the self (self-immolation) in the form of a 'victim' who or which represents the actual giver. This impulse to offer the self in sacrifice continues to this day. Numberless war-memorials carry the words 'Greater love hath no man than this, that a man lay down his life for his friends'. In agricultural communities man offered something that represented himself – something that was generally the result of his own labour in the fields, or, as in pastoral communities, the best animal in the herd with which the owner identified himself by laying his hand upon its head. But, we may ask, what are the psychological explanations of this offering of the self? Jung has pointed out[1] that the sacrificial gifts used in the Mass, bread and wine, in so far as they represent the products of human labour, stand for man himself. That which is materially offered in the Mass is a token that represents human life. Sacrifice by its very nature implies that the sacrificer is giving something that carries 'the marks of mineness'. Anything that a man makes or grows or captures is symbolically his 'self'. But this 'self' can have two meanings psychologically, according as to whether we accept the Freudian concept of the Super-Ego or that of the Jungian 'self'. Behind the ego that is influenced by public opinion, parental training and current moral codes (Freud's Super-Ego) there is, says Jung, a 'personality' of which man himself need not be aware. 'Just as a man still is what he always was, so he already is what he will become.' [2] This self which emerges in the course of individuation is different from the Super-Ego in that it is individual and not impersonal.

If a man offers a sacrifice for the sake of conforming to the prevailing social conventions then what he offers is not the self but his socially conditioned ego. But if he consciously obeys a feeling of compulsion to sacrifice his egocentric nature then he is offering that developing personality which is the self. The difference between these two sacrifices is that the first is an act of social piety which corresponds merely to 'going to Mass', the other to that devastating form of sacrifice which is most typically represented by Abraham offering his only son Isaac. If we attempt to look into Abraham's soul as he

[1] ***Psychology and Religion: West and East***: Collected Works: Vol. 11: section 4: 'The Psychology of the Mass'.

[2] Jung: op. cit. p. 258.

accepted the command to sacrifice his only son, what we see is a man who feels that what he is about to do is to plunge the knife into his own breast. Psychologically, Abraham was preparing to offer himself on that altar. He was about to be both priest and victim; the slayer and the slain. This psychological analysis reveals an aspect of the Mass which is not always consciously realized, although it is none the less always operative. What is offered in the Mass is not a fragment of pure wheaten bread and a mixture of water and wine, but a symbolical presentation of the flesh and blood, the life of the worshipper himself. Even as the Son of God offered himself to the Father, so man offers his own self.[1] Sacrificial death promotes life. 'He that loseth his life for my sake shall find it.'[2]

Jung explains this willingness to sacrifice the self as being due to the fact that man knows what it is to withdraw, to renounce, to accept suffering as the condition of subsequent triumph – transformation through self-immolation.[3] This view receives additional support from Emile Durkheim who held that the real greatness of man – whether primitive or civilized – is to be seen in the way he braves suffering.

> He never rises above himself with more brilliancy than when he subdues his own nature to the point of making it follow a way contrary to the use it would spontaneously take. . . . Suffering is the sign that certain of the bonds attaching him to his profane environment are broken: so it testifies that he is partially freed from his environment and, consequently, it is justly considered the instrument of deliverance. So he who is thus delivered is not the victim of a pure illusion when he believes himself invested with a sort of mastery over things, he really has raised himself above them by the very act of renouncing them. . . .[4]

The doctrine and practice of the Mass owe much of their psychological potency to the fact that the Mass itself is animated by the same impulses as have animated man for many thousands of years. This fact may be illustrated by referring to the close parallel between the Christian Mass and the Zoroastrian Haoma rite. Six centuries before Christ broke bread in the upper room, the prophet Zoroaster,

[1] This sacrifice of the self is significantly expressed in the Prayer of Oblation in the Communion Service of *The Book of Common Prayer*: 'And here we offer and present unto thee, O Lord, ourselves, our souls and bodies, to be a reasonable, holy and lively sacrifice unto thee; humbly beseeching thee, that, all we who are partakers of this Holy Communion, may be fulfilled with thy grace and heavenly benediction.'

[2] Matt. x. 39.

[3] See p. 114 *supra* re Ramakrishna: 'The sense of "I" in us is the greatest obstacle in the path of God-vision.'

[4] Durkheim: *Elementary Forms of the Religious Life* (1954) p. 315.

in his attempt to replace the polytheistic worship of the peoples of ancient Iran by a genuine monotheism, found it expedient to retain the ancient form of sacrifice known as the Haoma rite. This formerly was believed to be a means whereby man could have communion with a god. Now it could be the means of communion with the One True God. Haoma was both a plant and a god. As a plant it was gathered in mountainous districts and offered as a sacrifice.

> At the sacrificial ceremony it was 'slain' by being pounded in a mortar, and the juice that oozed out of it was consumed by priest and faithful as an elixir of immortality. As a god Haoma was the son of Ahura Mazdā the Wise Lord, and by Him he was established as the first priest of the cult of which he was himself, as plant, the victim. We thus have the strange spectacle of a son of God offering himself incarnate as a plant to his heavenly father. And the purpose of the sacrifice is to confer immortality on all who drink of the sacred liquid – the life-juice of a divine being pounded to death in a mortar. The god dies in his humble incarnate form in order to confer immortality on those who partake of the fluid which flows from him. As priest this strange god offers perpetual sacrifice to his father, and as victim, he enables man to participate in the very life of God.[1]

It is plain that despite the theological differences between the Christian explanation of the Mass and the Zoroastrian interpretation of the Haoma rite, the psychological motivation is substantially the same. All forms of sacrifice involve basic psychological motives; this is so whether it is the pattern of sacrifice described by Freud in *Totem and Taboo*, the human sacrifices of the Aztecs, those offered by agricultural and pastoral societies, the ancient Haoma rite or the Christian Mass. These motives are associated with two universally held beliefs – that sacrificial death promotes life, and that the highest sacrifice that man can offer to his God is his own self.

As an act of worship, sacrifice is one of the most impressive objectifications of symbolism known to mankind. It brings together into one combination the age-old archetypal imagery of the unconscious, the sense of the numinous, the impulse to self-abasement, the vocal expressions of joy and praise, and the universal tendency which man has to offer himself as victim for his own transformation. When these psychological functions co-operate as the expression of man's impulse to worship, it becomes clear that religion, in whatever form we may encounter it, is something more than a mere sublimation of instinctual libido.

[1] R. C. Zaehner: *At Sundry Times* (1958) pp. 152 ff.

Chapter XI

RELIGIOUS EXPERIENCE

There is, says Sir Frederic Bartlett,

> very wide agreement that religion, as a powerful influence in human life, has its foundation in some form of experience. . . . Experience is something which happens to an individual in so striking and remarkable a way that he can distinguish it from other things that happen to him, and can talk or write about it, or express it in one of the forms of art that human beings have discovered.[1]

Religious experience is not only something which stands out from the general background of our ordinary daily life, it is something of such a kind that the experient feels an inescapable compulsion to communicate and also to *explain* what happened to him. Such communications are attended by particular difficulties, partly because of the nature of the experience itself, and partly because of the limitations of human language – hence the existence of symbolism which enables man to express that which is logically inexpressible.

The nature of religious experience is such that although it affects the experient in a peculiarly personal way, it diminishes his self-awareness to such an extent that it enables him to enjoy that which all mystics have sought for, the transcendence of the human self in the Divine Self. Such experiences elude normal forms of description:

> It is notoriously difficult, or even impossible, to describe a sunset from memory. And the mystical vision is concerned with things more impalpable than a sunset, things which language was not framed to describe. . . Those who have had these experiences long to remember them and long to impart them. . . . But they must trust to their memory. The intellect is set to work and begins to schematize and set in order a vision which had no form and no parts . . . doubts, hesitations and reactions are forgotten. And often their narratives are unconsciously influenced by suggestion from outside; they have talked to directors, or they have read books. As a rule, the mystics have written their autobiographies

[1] F. C. Bartlett: *Religion as Experience, Belief, Action*: Riddell Memorial Lecture (1950) p. 5.

> when they were far advanced in their progress: their books are souvenirs and memoirs rather than journals. Teresa wrote her life in 1562 and 1566; but her 'mystical period' began in 1555. . . . We can judge how treacherous the memory of psychical states is when we compare Augustine's account of his conversion written many years after, in his *Confessions*, with the short and little treatises which he wrote at the time. . . .[1]

It is necessary to note not only that religious experiences are difficult both to describe and to remember, but that a distinction must be made between experiences which occur spontaneously (that is, involuntarily) and those which are deliberately sought for by means of personal disciplines. Some mystical insights appear to come to a man without his seeking for them, though an analysis of these involuntary experiences sometimes reveals the operation over many years of 'unconscious volition' – what Henri Poincaré called 'incubation'. But speaking generally, spontaneous religious experiences should be distinguished from those which come after long and often strenuous periods of physical and spiritual preparation. Such techniques are employed in most religions and we shall discuss some of them later in this chapter.

Motives

What we have now to ask is 'why do men deliberately seek for religious experiences?' The answer is twofold; it is because of something in the nature of man himself, and because of something in the nature of religion. Man is a creature who realizes to some degree the limitations of his own nature. He can never get rid of his mind, neither can he get rid of his body so long as he lives. Yet all the time he is wanting either to be rid of his body and to become a 'pure spirit' or else to be relieved of the embarrassment of a critical intelligence. Man pictured as Adam, a creature expelled from Paradise, is symbolically a 'true' picture. Man feels that he is a 'displaced person', restless, disappointed, without a home, always craving to return to some state of existence where he can be released from himself and the warring element of his nature.[2] This consciousness of an inner division and of

[1] W. R. Inge: *Personal Religion and the Life of Devotion* (1927) pp. 30–1.

[2] The opening passages in John Bunyan's *The Pilgrim's Progress* are among the most illuminating psychological descriptions of the nature of man. Man is a pilgrim seeking for a goal the way to which he does not know, conscious that he is carrying a great burden on his back. It is noteworthy that Bunyan should have presented his story in the form of a dream, for the real nature of man and his fundamental dissatisfactions can often be vividly revealed in this way.

a persistent but unspecified hunger is one of the chief characteristics which distinguish man as a 'religious' creature from the rest of the animal kingdom. Man always seems to have been aware of this interior disharmony, of a personal incompleteness which cannot be resolved by any of the normal psycho-physical activities of daily life. Always, even in religions like Buddhism, man seeks union with some Being or Power in contact with whom the disharmony of mind-and-body, matter-and-spirit, self-and-non-self, can be brought into a splendidly satisfying concordance. This yearning, which Professor Murphy calls 'man's essential quest', is the motivation behind all those techniques which are designed to create the conditions suitable for such religious experiences.

Religious Types and Attitudes

The matter may be carried a stage further by asking a vital question about the relationship of belief, preparatory techniques and experience itself. Does the fact that a man is a Christian, or a Buddhist, or practises Vedanta in any way affect the nature of such unifying experiences? It has been suggested that instead of dividing religious experiences into those which are Christian and those which are non-Christian, another classification might be more relevant – the distinction between *authoritarian* and *humanistic* forms of religion. The essential characteristic of all forms of authoritarian religion is that it demands the surrender of the individual to some power thought of as transcending the human person.[1] There are sound reasons for such an attitude. By voluntarily submitting to a higher authority man loses his sense of personal dissatisfaction and frustration, and by willingly associating himself with a Divine Power he achieves an exhilarating sense of fulfilment. In contrast to the authoritarian kind of religion, the humanistic type emphasizes the fact that the individual 'finds' himself by being in loving association with his fellows. Religious experience for the humanistic type is an experience which receives its significance from one's relationship with other men. The distinction between these two types of religion refers not only to the particular beliefs which men hold collectively but also to the individual's own psychological 'disposition'.

We are familiar with the distinction made by William James between the religion of what he called the 'sick soul' and the religion of the 'healthy-minded'. This is no pejorative classification but a

[1] See Erich Fromm: *Psycho-Analysis and Religion* (1951) p. 42 f.

distinction which applies as much to those who are Christians, Muhammadans, Hindus, Buddhists, as it does to those who belong to other religious allegiances. Human beings interpret their experiences not only in terms of belief but also in terms of their own personality, whether it be sick or healthy, introverted or extraverted.

> The constitutionally sombre religious person makes even of his religious peace a very sober thing. Danger still hovers in the air above it. Flexion and contraction are not wholly checked. It were sparrow-like and childish . . . to forget the imminent hawk on the bough. Lie low, rather, lie low: for you are in the hands of a living God. . . . If we turn to the sanguine onlooker, on the other hand, we find that deliverance is felt as incomplete unless the burden be altogether overcome and the danger forgotten. Such onlookers give us definitions that seem to the sombre minds of whom we have just been speaking to leave out all the solemnity that makes religious peace so different from merely animal joys. In the opinion of some writers an attitude might be called religious, though no touch were left in it of sacrifice or submission, no tendency to flexion, no bowing of the head. . . .[1]

Both attitudes are equally real and each has its own type of religious experience – every individual soul adopts to his God or the universe an attitude either of contraction and withdrawal, or else of expansion and joy. Many a young man or woman, for instance, brought up in an evangelical tradition with its insistence upon the necessity of conversion, has been brought to the point of despair by failing to recognize that he is by temperament and disposition a healthy-minded soul trying to behave as if he were a sick soul. Incompatibility between the attitude of some highly organized or doctrinally inflexible form of religion and that of some strongly temperamental individual, has frequently been a perplexing factor in the interpretation of religious experiences. But however strong the suggestions of the prevailing group attitude may be, the personal element in religious experience can never be ignored. Experience is highly individualistic, however much the subsequent description and explanation may be communally conditioned. For instance, the Augustinian canon, Walter Hilton (d. 1396), the author of *The Scale of Perfection*, laid great stress upon the personal factors in religion.

> Our holy Fathers here before taught us that *we should know the measure of our gift* and work upon that: not taking upon us by feigning more than we have in feeling . . . he that worketh in such grace as he hath, and

---

[1] William James: *Varieties of Religious Experience* (1928 edn) pp. 76–7.

> desireth by prayer meekly and lastingly after more, and after feeleth his heart stirred to follow the grace which he desired, he may safely run if he keep meekness. And, therefore, it is speedful that we know the gifts that are given to us of God, that we may work in them, for by these we shall be saved: as some by bodily works and deeds of mercy, some by great bodily penance, some by sorrow and weeping for their sins all their life-time, some by preaching and teaching, some by divers graces and gifts of devotion shall be saved and come to bliss.[1]

But Hilton proceeds to warn the reader that if he neglects his own particular gifts, and tries to imitate those of other men because they appear to him to be more 'fashionable' than his own, he will find after a time that he will draw the false conclusion that because his efforts at imitation have proved to be barren, therefore, the spiritual life is a fruitless pursuit. This advice applies to all men everywhere and to all forms of religious belief and practice, East and West. St Paul gives the same advice when writing to Timothy. 'Neglect not the gift that is in thee.'[2] All men have certain psychological functions in common, but individually we are not all of one type. Men of different temperaments have different spiritual abilities. It is important to remember this because rational criticisms of religious experiences are sometimes based upon the rather naïve assumption that since the critic himself has never had anything that resembles such experiences, therefore, the person who claims that he has is self-deceived, a charlatan or a sentimentalist. Some psycho-physical patterns render some men more sensitive to religious experience than others who have experiences of a different kind, or, possibly, may not be conscious of having had any such experience at all.

Experience and Temperaments

Dr W. H. Sheldon in *The Varieties of Temperament* (1942) has distinguished between three types of temperament and their religious affiliations. These three types are described as viscerotonic, somatotonic and cerebrotonic. Apparently no treatment can change these basic types; many men are a mixture of all three, but some belong almost entirely to one or other of these types. We have, therefore, to ask what these three types specify, and in what way they are related to religious experiences? Every religion has in it something that appeals to all three types, but certain aspects appeal more to one type than to

[1] Walter Hilton: *The Scale of Perfection*: ed. E. Underhill (1923) pp. 94–5.
[2] 1 Tim. iv. 14.

another, a fact that helps to explain why some people like the simplicity of a meeting of the Society of Friends and others the elaborate ceremonial of High Mass.

(1) The Viscerotonic temperament is associated with a physique which exhibits breadth of body, weight and a tendency to adipose tissue (endomorphic). Such a physique is often found with a character that is amiable, tolerant, slow to anger, dislikes solitude, desires company and companionship when in trouble, enjoys good family relationships, loves comfort and has an inclination to luxury.

(2) The Somatotonic temperament is found with a strong muscular body, an active and athletic physique often continuing from youth into active middle age (mesomorphic). Such physical development is generally associated with a character that is courageous, combative, loves danger, is indifferent to pain, dislikes being in enclosed places, can be ruthless when pursuing some objective, is strongly extraverted and when in personal trouble shows a tendency to seek some active occupation as a means of dispelling 'gloom and despondency'.

(3) The Cerebrotonic temperament is generally found with those whose physique is of a highly nervous type both in build and in gesture (ectomorphic). Such physiques tend to be like that of Shakespeare's Cassius who is described as having

. . . a lean and hungry look;
He thinks too much . . . he reads too much:
He is a great observer, and he looks
Quite through the deeds of men: he loves no plays . . .
Seldom he smiles and smiles in such a sort
As if he mock'd himself and scorned his spirit . . .[1]

Dr Sheldon's cerebrotonic type, whether it is exemplified by Cassius or not, tends to avoid company, is emotionally restrained, dislikes open spaces, is introverted and when in trouble needs solitude.

Each of these three types has its own religious orientation.[2] The viscerotonic type inclines to sacramentalism, with solemn and elaborate worship in magnificent architectural settings. Because of his love of family relationships the cult of the Divine Mother and Child often figures prominently in his religious devotions. The somatotonic type shows a strong inclination to make converts, a readiness to

[1] *Julius Caesar*: I. ii. 197.

[2] A comparison of the religious pictures which great artists have painted would reveal an interesting correlation between their choice and treatment of subject-matter and their own temperaments and physiques.

suffer martyrdom as well as to persecute others for 'a good cause'. This type has a marked tendency to austerity, and a dogmatic insistence upon morality and good works rather than upon sacraments and rituals. We need to notice that when those who belong to this type become aware of their interior life, such knowledge often comes to them as a violent revelation, as an overwhelming conversion, so that they throw themselves into the service of their newly found faith with a vigour that corresponds to their strong physique. But our third type, the cerebrotonic, is associated with a very different religious attitude. Being introvert, the cerebrotonic type lives inside himself, rather than in the outside world. The revelations of religion, or for that matter, of psycho-analysis, have for him no specially disturbing message, because he has always lived within himself. Such a type rarely experiences that convulsive kind of emotional experience that is so characteristic of somatotonic temperaments. The positive contribution of the cerebrotonic type is often made in the contemplative life. Psychologically, the history of mysticism is mainly the record of the cerebrotonic temperament, not that this temperament in itself produces mystical experiences but such experiences are most readily apprehended by those who have this particular temperament. This type often renounces, or seeks to avoid, ritualistic forms of worship as impediments to the soul's free encounter with the Divine. As compared with the viscerotonic type which, when it takes to religion, relinquishes possessions and personal luxuries, transferring them to religion and its forms of worship, the cerebrotonic type regards the life of voluntary poverty as the most natural form of life, while he worships in churches almost devoid of ornament. Architecturally the churches of the Cistercians and the Carthusians are very austerely decorated compared with those which house Benedictine and other monastic Orders.[1] It is the cerebrotonics who design special systems of religious exercises both as aids to private devotion and also as means to mystical experience. Systems such as those which stem from Shankara, the Hindu sage who was active in Southern India towards the end of the eighth century A.D.,[2] or from Plotinus who has been

[1] For descriptions of modern Cistercian monastic houses and their exercises see Thomas Merton: *The Waters of Silence* (1950), and Patrick Leigh Fermor: *A Time to Keep Silence* (1957) chap. II: 'From Solesmes to La Grande Trappe'.

[2] Shankara, who died at the age of thirty-two, was responsible for an enormous religious output, including some of the most brilliant and learned commentaries on the Upanishads, the Brahma-sutras and the Bhagavad-Gītā: see Radhakrishnan: *Indian Philosophy* (1927) Vol. I.

called 'the father of Christian mysticism', or from Meister Eckhart, the Dominican friar who in the fourteenth century initiated the German 'school' of mysticism – all these systems, both East and West, are derived from men of cerebrotonic temperaments.

Attempts have been made, perhaps somewhat arbitrarily, to classify the great religions of the world in terms of these temperamental types. The religions of Vedic India in their use of ritual and their mystical practices are said to be a combination of the viscerotonic and cerebrotonic types, showing considerable tolerance of other religions and exhibiting little tendency to proselytization. In China, Confucianism seems to be predominantly viscerotonic, a religion of forms and ceremonials with a strong bias in favour of the Family. Muhammadanism is a somatotonic religion, hard and militant with a strong zeal for making converts, inflicting persecution and a readiness for martyrdom. Christianity is a mixture of all three types. It has ritualistic and aesthetic aspects which correspond to the viscerotonic type; contemplative and mystical aspects which correspond to the cerebrotonic, and, more recently, a devotion to the social aspects of the Gospel which corresponds to the somatotonic temperament. But whatever a man's temperament may be, no religion makes a full appeal to him unless it indicates some way by which he may experience what is believed to be an authentic commerce between man and the Ultimate. It is in their pursuit of the Ultimate that certain temperaments have played such a notable part in religion, especially in those practices and experiences which are labelled mystical.

Mystical Phenomena

This brief discussion of the relationship of temperament and religion has been pursued for a definite purpose. Psychologically, it has often been objected that religious experiences are not related to Ultimate Reality but are the product of abnormal personalities. Evelyn Underhill, in her several works on Mysticism, agrees that many of the experiences ascribed to saints and mystics (as well as to lesser men) are difficult to accept on *strictly rational grounds*. The fact that religious experiences so often seem to be associated with such psychical phenomena as visions, auditions, automatic scripts, levitation and so forth, is often a ground for adverse criticism. Pierre Janet, for instance, once objected that the kind of things said to occur in the lives of medieval saints and mystics suggests that these men and women would, if they were living today, be patients in mental hospitals. Rufus Jones, a much more sympathetic interpreter, whose *Studies in Mystical Religion* is a classic, says that many people find, for instance, the statement that St Francis of Assisi bore on his body the stigmata of the Crucifixion, evidence of the saint's abnormal personality. But this physical occurrence need not be a ground for dismissing the spiritual validity of the saint's experiences.

> For weeks he [Francis] had been going over in his thoughts the memories of Calvary. His Bible opened itself to the story of Christ's passion. The love and suffering of Jesus had burned themselves into his heart. He had, too, been fasting for weeks, and the thought of the approaching feast of the Exaltation of the Cross was constantly before his mind. He had spent the entire night in prayer – September 14th 1224 – when a vision came to him with the rising sun:
>
> 'A seraph with outspread wings flew towards him from the edge of the horizon, and bathed his soul in raptures unutterable. In the centre of the vision appeared a cross, and the seraph was nailed upon it. When the vision disappeared, he felt sharp sufferings mingled with ecstasy in the first moments. Stirred to the very depths of his being, he was anxiously asking the meaning of it all, when he perceived upon his body the Stigmata of the Crucified.' [1]

The mystical experiences of St Paul and of that formidable mystic St Teresa are sometimes held to be due to epilepsy or hysteria; indeed, there are those who treat all religious experiences which are accompanied by abnormal psycho-physical phenomena as being the result of unhealthy psychological personalities.[2]

On the other hand, many of the pious make the opposite mistake of supposing that auditions and similar phenomena are attestations of the genuineness of mystical occurrences. This type of piety is as materialistic in its insistence upon physical wonders as those forms of scepticism which attempt to explain spiritual events in purely materialistic terms. It may well be doubted whether St Anthony of Padua, a younger contemporary of St Francis, did actually hold the Infant Christ in his arms, or whether the Holy Ghost really told the Blessed Angela of Foligno that 'he loved her better than any other woman in the Vale of Spoleto'.[3] Piety of this order seeks to elevate

[1] Rufus Jones: op. cit. pp. 164 ff. The fact that St Francis had for many weeks been mentally concentrating upon the Crucifixion lends support to the suggestion, made earlier in this chapter, that an analysis of some involuntary religious experiences reveals the operation over a long time of some unconscious volition, the incubation of some dominant theme or idea.

[2] Evelyn Underhill discusses this at some length in *Mysticism* (1945 edn) pp. 266 ff.

[3] See Evelyn Underhill: op. cit. p. 267.

the hallucinatory to the status of a Beatific Vision.[1] Too many of the accounts of religious experience have been decorated with sensory inventions, sweet smells, sensations of touch and burning, but such things are all capable of a psychological explanation, and it is noteworthy that the great mystics have warned others against attaching too much importance to these secondary matters. But we must not dismiss them all as merely pious inventions. For instance, stigmatization is by no means restricted to mystical experiences. It has been explained as a form of *dermographism* in which 'an image existing in the subject's mind becomes outlined on the skin'. Baudouin cites a case from Charles Richet:

> A mother is watching her child at play. Accidentally the child unfastens the catch suspending a heavy sliding door in front of the fire-place, and it is in danger of being guillotined. The mother's heart leaps to her mouth, and then, in a moment, there forms round her neck – the threatened part of the child – a raised erythematous circle, a weal that endures for several hours. Here we have a striking instance of the power of emotion.[2]

Baudouin then proceeds to give modern examples of what he calls 'spontaneous stigmatization' where accurate observations have been made in cases of sphygmographic tracing, where the circulation of the blood has been directly controlled by auto-suggestion on religious subjects so that the body of the experient is marked by such tracings as those of the Crucifixion. These stigmatizations are not restricted to Christian forms of mysticism but are to be found in other religions.

> It would be an error to look upon them as, in essence, manifestations of an exceptional or morbid temperament. We need not go to religious devotees or to persons suffering from grave hysteria, when we are looking for instances in which suggestion leads to organic modifications. . . . We

---

[1] Dr W. R. Inge observed that 'in the mysticism of the Cloister . . . mystical theology came to be closely connected with strange stories of supernatural visitations which the modern psychologist can only regard as signs of mental disturbance. . . . They are undoubtedly a genuine experience but it is equally certain that they have no objective reality and that they are not wholesome.' *Personal Religion and the Life of Devotion* (1927) p. 23.

Gerald Bullett observes on the same matter that the accounts given by many mystics seem to be so pathological and sensuously erotic that it is not surprising that some psychological writers reject the validity of such experiences. But 'it would be unwise to reject illumination because we do not care for the design of the lamp shade'. *The English Mystics* (1950) p. 19.

[2] Charles Baudouin: *Suggestion and Auto-suggestion* (1920) p. 100.

have to note that there is no radical difference between the action of suggestion when its results are purely functional and its action when its results are organic. If we admit that suggestion can act in the former cases (and this has long been admitted) there need be no difficulty about acknowledging the reality of its action in the latter cases.[1]

Such examples support the view that stigmatizations may be historical events, that they are not necessarily the result of morbid personalities, and also that their occurrence is by no means to be interpreted as the 'hall-mark' of spirituality. It cannot, however, be denied that some of these psycho-physical phenomena are in fact the results of morbidity, some are signs of incipient insanity and all have borrowed something from the temperamental peculiarities of the persons to whom such phenomena have occurred. Furthermore, the pictorial content of mystical visions is determined to a large extent by the theological beliefs of their experients. No Buddhist ever had a vision of the Blessed Virgin Mary, and St Benedict never saw a vision of the Blessed Goddess Kwan-Yin. The point is that these 'theologically artistic' visions *are not in themselves the real experience*, they are the means whereby the real element in the experience is clothed in forms appropriate to the religious allegiance of each particular mystic.[2] The reality to which they refer is of greater importance than either their pictorial presentation or the psycho-physical phenomena which accompany the belief of the experient. None the less we need some criteria whereby we may be able to distinguish between a valid experience and a pathological or hallucinatory occurrence.

Mystical Criteria

In the first place there is the testimony of the person who has had the experience – his feeling of utter convincingness. From the rational point of view, an hallucination can give rise to the same degree of

[1] Charles Baudouin: op. cit. pp. 101–2.

[2] This is the same point as is made by Miss Sackville-West in her study of St Teresa of Avila. 'Is it, or is it not conceivable that in the hypothetical case of a person who had never heard of God, Christ, the Communion of Saints, the Devil, or any of the accepted appurtenances of religion, the phenomenon of divine visions or loculations should occur? Is it possible to imagine our Lady appearing to one who was unacquainted with the story of Christ's nativity? Is it possible to imagine a stigmatist to whom the story of the Crucifixion should be totally unknown? If such cases exist, proven beyond suspicion, they would seem to settle the matter once and for all; but in their absence it would seem logical to conclude that the phenomena of mystical theology must take their origin from some image already in the mind.' *The Eagle and the Dove* (1943).

conviction as does a religious experience but a religious experience, unlike an hallucination, is something that is related to a man's whole life.

> If you have intuitions at all, they come from a deeper level of your nature than the loquacious level which rationalism inhabits. Your whole subconscious life, your impulses, your faith, your needs, your divinations, have prepared the premises, of which your consciousness now feels the weight of the result; and something in you absolutely *knows* that that result must be truer than any logic-chopping rationalistic talk, however clever, that may contradict it.[1]

It is when we turn to enumerate the general characteristics of religious experience that we find ourselves on more conclusive grounds. Broadly speaking those who have had religious experiences seem to agree that (1) the visible world is not all there is; (2) the true 'end' of man is union with some other Self than the human self; (3) such an experience endows daily life with a certain lyrical quality and a sense of purpose and courage that it lacked before; (4) those who have had such experiences enjoy 'the assurance of ultimate safety in the midst of imminent peril'; (5) the last criterion is found in the after-effects of the vision itself. A transcendental element seems to have been present whenever an experience is followed by some life-enhancing quality which affects other persons for their spiritual good.

These seem to be the broad characteristics of religious experience whether these experiences are of a spontaneous kind or subsequent to a prolonged discipline. For those who find these explanations rationally unacceptable, there is this declaration which may satisfy many who are aware of the 'determinism' of their own particular psychological pattern:

> If we cannot find God in your house or in mine, upon the roadside or the margin of the sea; in the bursting seed or the opening flower; in the day duty or the night musing; in the general laugh and the secret grief; in the procession of life, ever entering afresh, and solemnly passing by and dropping off; I do not think we should discern him any more on the grass of Eden, or beneath the moonlight of Gethsemane.[2]

This quotation confronts us with the necessity of considering yet another aspect of mysticism.

[1] William James: *Varieties*: p. 73.

[2] James Martineau: *Endeavours after a Christian Life*: quoted James: op. cit. p. 475.

Nature Mysticism and Mysticism Proper

A classical definition of mysticism is to be found in Professor E. G. Browne's *A Year among the Persians.*

> There is hardly any soil, be it ever so barren, where it [mysticism] will not strike root; hardly any creed, however stern, however formal, round which it will not twine itself. It is indeed the eternal cry of the human soul for rest; the insatiable longing of a being wherein infinite ideals are fettered and cramped by a miserable actuality; and so long as man is less than an angel and more than a beast, this cry will not for the moment fail to make itself heard. Wonderfully uniform, too, is its tenor; in all ages, in all countries, in all creeds, whether it come from the Brahmin sage, the Greek philosopher, the Persian poet, or the Christian quietist, it is in essence an enunciation more or less clear, more or less eloquent, of the aspiration of the soul to cease altogether from self, and to be at one with God.[1]

There are many writers on mysticism who, like Professor E. G. Browne, assume that mysticism is basically one and the same all over the world, and that in whatever religion it is found man has the same impulse 'to cease altogether from self and to be at one with God'. The present writer shares this view, but there are substantial grounds for objection. Professor R. C. Zaehner insists that it is necessary to distinguish between nature mysticism, which is one of the most common forms of mystical experience, and those kinds which appear to give a 'direct' apprehension of the Being of God. Nature mysticism is a form of experience in which one ceases from self, but this, says Professor Zaehner, does not necessarily achieve union with God. Here, for example, is an experience of the great English naturist, Richard Jefferies:

> I was utterly alone with the sun and the earth. Lying down on the grass, I spoke in my soul to the earth, the sun, the air, and the distant sea far beyond sight. I thought of the earth's firmness – I felt it bear me up; through the grassy couch there came an influence as if I could feel the great earth speaking to me. I thought of the wandering air – its pureness, which is its beauty; the air touched me and gave me something of itself. I spoke to the sea; though so far, in my mind I saw it, green at the rim of the earth and blue in deeper ocean; I desired to have its strength, its mystery and glory. Then I addressed the sun, desiring the soul equivalent of his light and brilliance, his endurance and unwearied race. I turned to the blue heaven over, gazing into its depths, inhaling its exquisite colour and sweetness. The rich blue of the unattainable flower of the sky drew

---

[1] E. G. Browne: op. cit. (3rd edn 1950) p. 136. See also Margaret Smith: *An Introduction to the History of Mysticism* (1930).

my soul towards it, and there it rested, for pure colour is rest of heart. By all these I prayed; I felt an emotion of the soul beyond all definition; prayer is a puny thing to it, and the word is a rude sign to the feeling, but I know no other.

By the blue heaven, by the rolling sun bursting through untrodden space, a new ocean of ether every day unveiled . . . then, I prayed by the sweet thyme, whose little flowers I touched with my hand; by the slender grass; by the crumble of dry chalky earth I took up and let fall through my fingers. Touching the crumble of earth, the blade of grass, the thyme flower, breathing the earth-encircling air, holding out my hand for the sunbeams to touch it, prone on the sward in token of deep reverence, thus I prayed that I might touch to the unutterable existence infinitely higher than deity.[1]

This is but one of many such passages in *The Story of my Heart*. It comes as a surprise to know that Jefferies emphatically denied that these experiences had anything to do with theistic belief. Deeply 'mystical' in his appreciation of Nature, Jefferies was completely non-theistic in his interpretations of such experiences. Yet he somehow envisages 'matter ennobled and sanctified by spirit'.[2] Jefferies refers to 'the unutterable existence infinitely higher than deity' [3] and seems to have believed that Nature was pervaded by 'a subtle power' which could produce a sympathetic response in those who were sensitive to such an influence. The religions of Vedic India, as we have seen, included a concept of *prāna* which seems to have been of the same order as Jefferies's 'vital force'. Indeed, it corresponds to the all-pervading 'breath' which for primitive man gave rise to the concept of soul or psyche. Jefferies, without apparently realizing it, by his reference to 'the existence infinitely higher than deity' was not so much repudiating the Christian concept of deity, as agreeing with St Thomas Aquinas, for whom the concept of deity was 'the purest form of ideas'.[4]

If in our religious experiences we have a sense of being *en rapport* with the infinite horizon, with the life of the far-stretching hills and the heaving ocean, we may be pantheists but not necessarily theists.

[1] Richard Jefferies: *The Story of my Heart* (Kingsway Classics: no date) pp. 6–9.

[2] Zaehner: *Mysticism – Sacred and Profane* (1957) p. 49.

[3] On the theological side we need to notice a point made by Paul Tillich who uses the phrase 'the God above God'. God who is above God is present, though hidden, in every divine-human encounter. 'If God encounters man, God is neither object nor subject and is, therefore, above the scheme into which theism has forced him.' See Paul Tillich: *The Courage to Be* (1962) pp. 180 ff.

[4] Zaehner: op. cit. p. 48.

For a mystical experience to be genuine (from the Christian point of view) it must achieve a sense of union with God thought of as distinct from the realm of Nature, although Nature has often been the means whereby the soul has come to have union with God. An experience will illustrate this point. A letter written by J. Estlin Carpenter, from North Wales, when he was a young man in Oxford and in a condition of religious apathy, tells of one such experience.

> I went out one afternoon for a walk alone. I was in the empty unthinking state in which one saunters along country lanes, simply yielding oneself to the casual sights around which give a town-bred lad with country yearnings such intense delight. Suddenly I became conscious of the presence of some one else. I cannot describe it, but I felt that I had as direct a perception of God all round about me as I have of you when we are together. It was no longer a matter of inference, it was an immediate act of spiritual (or whatever adjective you like to employ) apprehension. It came unsought, absolutely unexpectedly. I remember the wonderful transfiguration of the far-off woods and hills as they seemed to blend in the infinite being with which I was thus brought into relation. This experience did not last long. But it sufficed to change all my feeling. I had not found God because I had never looked for him. But he had found me. . . . The sense of a direct relation to God then generated in my soul has become a part of my habitual thought and feeling.[1]

It may be argued that nature mysticism is not the same as theistic mysticism, but the person having such an experience may be led to a deeper union with God whether thought of as distinct from Nature or not.

Mystical Techniques

As we have seen, the natural world can sometimes furnish men with a taking-off point for a transcendental experience, but other men have regarded Nature as that which hinders their attempts to achieve union with the transcendental. As a consequence of this belief, men for centuries have attempted to devise methods whereby they could make the opaqueness of material things so 'thin' that Reality might be perceived if only 'through a glass darkly'. Today we understand the medical aspects of many of these techniques much more accurately than did the mystics themselves. Their knowledge of such techniques was a purely pragmatic one – they found that by doing or refraining from doing certain things, particular results followed.

Instead of illustrating this argument with much-quoted examples

[1] C. H. Herford: *Joseph Estlin Carpenter* (1929) pp. 9–10.

taken from medieval Christian mysticism, we may select one of the most famous examples of mysticism in the East as it is described by Dr W. Y. Evans-Wentz.[1] In his Introduction, Evans-Wentz gives some personal details of Jetsün Milarepa: 'This *Biography* of one of the Great Religious Geniuses of our human race presents to us a vivid record of the social conditions which prevailed in the Tibet of the 11th and 12th centuries of the Christian era.' Milarepa tells how he entered into prolonged meditation in the Mountain Solitudes:

> I set forth . . . and came to the Dragkar-Taso Cave . . . where having provided myself with a hard mattress seat and spreading my bedding upon it, I took the vows of not descending to any village or human habitation. . . . Having thus vowed I sang this song [prayer] consecrating my vows:
>
> *Offspring of Naropa and of the Saving Path,*
> *May [I] the hermit cling successfully to solitude.*
>
> *May pleasures of the world illusory not tempt me;*
> *But may Tranquillity of Meditation be increased;*
>
> *May I not lie steeped in Unconsciousness of Quietude,*
> *But may the Blossom of the Superconsciousness bloom forth in me.*
>
> *May various mind-created worldly thoughts not vex me:*
> *But may the foliage luxuriant, of Uncreatedness, burst forth in me.*
>
> *May I, in Hermitage, be troubled not with mental conflict;*
> *But may I ripen fruit of Knowledge and Experience . . .*
>
> This prayer finished, I continued my meditations, living on just a little flour mixed with whatever food came in my way. I mentally acquired knowledge of the *Mahā-Mudrā* [Great Symbol]; but my body, being too weak, was unable to control the Airs [psycho-physical nervous power or fluid] of my system, so that I did not acquire the Ecstatic Internal Warmth, and continued to be very sensitive to the cold. . . .[2]

Later, Milarepa was able to practise 'the three exercises of Physical, Vocal and Mental Culture, and developed the Ecstatic Physical Warmth . . . and continued my meditations for over three years, both night and day, and I could feel my spiritual knowledge expanding and improving greatly. . . .' Upon one occasion, he left his cave and

> strolled forth . . . discovering a sunny spot with good springs of water, with plenty of nettles growing round about . . . living on nettle broth

[1] See *Tibet's Great Yogi – Milarepa* (1928).

[2] op. cit. pp. 193–4.

> alone, I continued my meditations. I had no clothes on the outside of my body, nor any wholesome food inside. My body became shrunken to a mere skeleton; and it was greenish in hue, just like the nettle, and over it grew a covering of greenish hair.[1]

This state of affairs continued for years during which Milarepa, faithful to his vows, sought for the final attainment of Nirvāna by resisting all connexions with the *sangsāric* (worldly) life. At last after having 'undergone very severe trials and penances imposed by his *Guru* Marpa, he eventually enters upon the Path of Light; and eventually reaches in the words of the narrative "the greatest of all great successes that can ever fall to the lot of mortal man" '.[2] There are points of immediate relevance in this excerpt. The first is in the prayer with which Milarepa consecrated his vows, where he prays that he may not 'lie steeped in Unconsciousness of Quietude'. Unconsciousness in itself does not necessarily lead to Enlightenment, although we have seen that Jung held the transcendental elements of religious experience come to us through the unconscious. Some distinction must be made between the state of suspended animation or '*yogically* induced hibernation' which many yogis claim to have achieved, sometimes for periods of many years, and other states of psychological unconsciousness. We may note that Buddhist yogis condemn all forms of torpor since the vow not to sleep for any length of time is one of the twelve accepted austerities of Buddhist mystical practice.

A second point of interest is Milarepa's reference to his inability at one time to control what he calls 'the Airs'. Here we have a reference to the word *Vāyu* which is derived from the Sanskrit word *Va* (meaning to breathe) which has the same psychological significance as *prāna*, the life-force which is in so many languages the same concept as 'soul' or 'breath of life'. M. Jacques Bacot, in his version of Milarepa's *Biography*, refers in some detail to this aspect of Milarepa's discipline.

> Then, in the squatting posture [*āsana*] which resembleth the 'six Internal Hearths', I sought the well-being of my body. By means of the condition of the breathing which giveth regularity, I sought rightness of speech. By the condition of mine own liberation which controlleth the imagination, I sought calmness of mind. After that I entered into meditation. Soon the internal heat began to come over me.[3]

---

[1] ibid. [2] op. cit. p. 3.
[3] Jacques Bacot: abridged trans. *Milarepa: Biography*: Paris (1925).

Here again we see the part which breathing plays in meditation. An extensive literature is now available in the West which shows that the various practices associated with Yoga use systems of mental control for breathing and the postures of the body. The aim of such exercises is the same as that which animates Western forms of mystical discipline, union with Deity, whether that union be with the Buddha of Nirvāna, Brahmā or the Incarnate Christ as the Bridegroom. The word *yoga* itself testifies to this motivation, since the root *yuj* means 'to join'.

From this brief excursus into oriental mystical techniques we now turn to an interesting contemporary experiment in the West, and its yet more interesting explanation.

A Contemporary Experiment

In two small books, Aldous Huxley has given an account of certain experiments which he made with the drug known as *mescalin.*[1] The importance of these experiments lies not so much in the actual processes employed as in Huxley's reflections upon the use of these techniques, for Huxley shows how difficult it is to distinguish between these mescalin experiments and experiences which are generally accepted as genuinely mystical. Yet it is one thing to induce psychophysical effects such as are commonly associated with mystical experiences, and another to have an actual mystical experience. The subject is one which it is difficult to elucidate psychologically, but in view of Huxley's experiments it calls for serious attention.

It is known that such processes as hypnosis, the flashing of a stroboscopic lamp or the introduction of certain drugs into the blood stream can affect our normal consciousness. Huxley experimented, as others have done, with a drug which has a powerful effect upon the brain, and hence upon consciousness. It appears that early Spanish explorers in Mexico and the American South-West found that the Indians ate a root called *peyotl* which they venerated as though it were divine.[2] Chemical analysis has found that this root contains a drug known to us as *mescalin.* The cult of Peyotism is still practised by native American Indians in such areas as Texas and Wisconsin, a

[1] Aldous Huxley: *The Doors of Perception* (1954) and *Heaven and Hell* (1956) published together in a Penguin edn (1959). For a medical discussion of mescalin see Mayer-Gross, Slater and Roth: *Clinical Psychiatry* (1954) pp. 361 ff.

[2] Cf., with what we have already said about the Zoroastrian attitude to the *haoma* plant.

cult which has been 'baptized' into Christianity among the members of the Native American Church, which is an indigenous religious movement which originated in the south-west of America.[1] At a sacramental meal small slices of this sacred root are eaten, and participants then pass into a 'mystical' condition which lasts for several hours. The sacramental use of this drug appears to be motivated by the same desire as the disciplines of medieval mystics and oriental yogis, a desire to be lifted out of the rut of ordinary perception and to be shown for a few timeless moments the outer and the inner world *sub specie aeternitatis*. If 'the doors of perception' are cleansed, or opened just a little wider, the finite world appears in its proper light – the infinite. Something of this wider perception was brilliantly expressed by the Welsh mystical writer, Thomas Traherne, who in *Centuries of Meditation* said: 'Your enjoyment of the world is never right until every morning you awake in Heaven, see yourself in your Father's Palace, and look upon the skies, the earth and air as celestial joys, having such a reverend esteem of them as if you were among the angels . . .' Huxley describes how 'the doors of his perception' were opened when he took four-tenths of a gramme of mescalin dissolved in half a glass of water and sat down to wait for the results. The experience lasted several hours, and Huxley and an observer recorded their conversation on a tape-recording machine. This is how it began:

> I took my pill at eleven. An hour and a half later I was sitting in my study, looking intently at a small glass vase. The vase contained only three flowers – a full-blown Belle of Portugal rose, shell pink with a hint at every petal's base of hotter, flamier hue; a large magenta and cream-coloured carnation; and, pale purple at the end of its broken stalk, the bold heraldic blossom of an iris. . . . At breakfast that morning I had been struck by the lively dissonance of its colours. But that was no longer the point. I was not looking now at an unusual flower arrangement. I was seeing what Adam had seen on the morning of the creation – the miracle, moment by moment, of naked existence.

---

[1] A highly informative account of this sacramental use of peyotl among members of this Native Church is to be found in an article by Dr Humphry Osmond (who is the author of *The Chemical Basis of Clinical Psychiatry* with Dr Abram Hoffer) entitled 'That Night in the Tepi' in the Autumn (1961) issue of *The Twentieth Century*: Vol. CLXX. No. 1011. pp. 38 ff. Dr Ruth Benedict gives a detailed account of the use of the fermented juice of the giant cactus by Mexican Indians, of the datura or jimson weed by tribes in Southern California, and the brewing of cactus beer by the Pima, all as means of inducing 'religious intoxication'. *Patterns of Culture* (1946) pp. 61 ff.

'Is it agreeable?' somebody asked. . . . 'Neither agreeable nor disagreeable,' I answered. 'It just *is.*' *Istigkeit* – wasn't that the word Meister Eckhart liked to use? 'Is-ness' . . . My eyes travelled from the rose to the carnation, and from that feathery incandescence to the smooth scrolls of sentient amethyst which were the iris. The Beatific Vision, *Sat Chit Ananda,* Being-Wareness-Bliss – for the first time I understood, not on the verbal level, not by inchoate hints or at a distance, but precisely and completely what those prodigious syllables referred to. And then I remembered a passage I had read in one of Suzuki's essays. 'What is the Dharma-Body of the Buddha?' (The Dharma-Body of the Buddha is another way of saying, Mind, Suchness, the Void, the Godhead.) The question is asked in a Zen monastery by an earnest and bewildered novice. And with the prompt irrelevance of one of the Marx Brothers, the Master answers, 'The hedge at the bottom of the garden!' 'And the man who realizes this truth,' the novice dubiously enquires, 'what, may I ask, is he?' Groucho gives him a whack over the shoulders with his staff and answers, 'A golden-haired lion.'

It had been, when I read it, only a vaguely pregnant piece of nonsense. Now it was all as clear as day. . . . Of course the Dharma-Body of the Buddha was the hedge at the bottom of the garden. At the same time, and no less obviously, it was these flowers, it was anything that I, or rather the blessed Not-I released for a moment from my throttling embrace – cared to look at. . . .

The description goes on to say how Huxley looked at the coloured books on the shelves of his study walls, how like the flowers they glowed with brighter colours: 'Red books like rubies: emerald books; books bound in white jade: books of agate, of aquamarine; of yellow topaz: lapis lazuli books. . . .' But Huxley looked at them not in terms of their place or distance but in a context to which three-dimensional description was no longer applicable. 'The mind was primarily concerned, not with measures and locations, but with being and meaning.' And this indifference to space was accompanied by an even greater indifference to time.[1]

The rest of Huxley's description is equally vivid, but the question soon begins to intrude itself into our reading, what are the *chemical* facts behind this curious enlargement of perception, this seeing of the finite in 'the light that never was, on sea or land'? The activity of the brain is to a large extent dependent upon an adequate supply of glucose to the brain cells. Mescalin and a number of other drugs reduce the amount of glucose in the blood that passes over the brain, with the result that the phenomenal world appears to be different to the person into whose blood stream the drug has been introduced. The

[1] Aldous Huxley: *The Doors of Perception* (1954) pp. 12 ff.

ego is no longer troubled about the world of space and time; it is interested instead in a realm of intense colour and light, and has a feeling of identity with a world in which *being* is felt to be identified with the All.[1]

It could be objected that these artificially induced experiences have no more relevance to Ultimate Reality than the 'pictures' which patients see when emerging from anaesthetics. Huxley deals with these objections against 'artificially induced Paradises', by saying that 'most men and women lead lives at the worst so painful, at the best, so monotonous, poor and limited, that the urge to escape, the longing to transcend themselves if only for a few moments, is and always has been one of the principal appetites of the soul'.[2] Here, in the West, for the greater part of the population, alcohol, tobacco and, more recently, bromides, barbiturates and the like are what H. G. Wells once called in a revealing phrase 'doors in the Wall' which, when opened, reveal to us a paradise from which many men are most of their lives firmly extruded. The fact that the Western world spends more on tobacco and alcohol than it does on education may be due to the yearning of the self to escape, if only for the length of time that it takes to smoke a cigarette or to drink one whisky, from the world of everyday drabness, as well as from the discordant strifes within one's own consciousness. But when this has been admitted, we should not fail to observe that in Buddhist literature, the use of all such stimulants, including even such common narcotics as strong tea and coffee, are held to be deleterious by exciting the nerves which control the 'animal' in man's nature, thus inhibiting the elevating influence of the psyche or soul.[3] Professor Zaehner strongly criticized Huxley's suggestion that drug-induced experiences could have the same significance as those experienced by acknowledged mystics. But such objections are two-edged.

If drugs produce experiences which seem to be pseudo-transcendental in character then the experiences which follow the self-inflicted tortures of ascetics, Christian and non-Christian alike, are by the same token, open to the same objection. There is psychologically and chemically very little difference between taking a drug and submitting oneself to such masochistic mortifications as those endured

[1] Cf. these experiences with Professor Zaehner's who whilst under the influence of this drug visited the cathedral of Christ Church, Oxford: *Mysticism Sacred and Profane*: Appendix B. pp. 212 ff.

[2] op. cit. p. 49.

[3] Cp. Evans-Wentz: op. cit. p. 191 fn. 1.

over many years by the Blessed Suso, except that the former is pleasant and the latter horrifyingly painful.[1] The nervous system is always being affected chemically. When the Lenten fast is observed with strictness for forty days, the chemistry of the body is strongly affected. Many of the most vivid visions of the medieval mystics seem to have occurred during periods of prolonged fasting. When ascetic practices include such mortifications as flagellation the effect of such beating is 'the equivalent of fairly extensive surgery without anaesthetics'.[2] As a result large quantities of histamine and adrenalin are released into the blood stream and when, as usually happens among ascetics, the self-inflicted wounds begin to fester, they release other toxins which further affect the action of the brain. On a purely chemical basis, it could be argued that mystical insights which appear to be associated with alterations of the chemistry of the body are not essentially different from the insights which it is claimed can be experienced by the administration of drugs. Are we then to conclude that all experiences associated with the use of external aids are to be dismissed as invalid or hallucinatory?

That question implies too much, and admits too little. The plain fact is that all human experiences, whether religious or not, are accompanied by chemical changes. If we talk about an experience as being *purely* aesthetic, *purely* intellectual, *purely* emotional or *purely* spiritual, we are betraying the fact that we have never fully appreciated the part that biochemistry plays at every moment of human exist-

[1] The practices of American and Mexican Indians exhibit much the same characteristics as those of Christian ascetics. Long and painful means were used in order to induce supernatural visions. We notice, too, that much the same techniques of concentration were employed as those used by Christian mystics. 'On the western plains men sought their visions with hideous tortures. They cut strips from the skin of their arms, they struck off fingers, they swung themselves from tall poles by straps inserted under the muscles of their shoulders. They went without food and water for extreme periods. They sought in every way to achieve an order of experience set apart from daily living. . . . Sometimes they stood motionless, their hands tied behind them, or they staked out a tiny spot from which they could not move till they had received blessing. . . . At all events a man went alone, or, if he was seeking his vision by torture and someone had to go out with him to tie him to the pole from which he was to swing till he had his supernatural experience, his helper did his part and left him alone for his ordeal. It was necessary to keep one's mind fixed upon the expected visitation. Concentration was the technique above all others upon which they relied. "Keep thinking it all the time," the old medicine men said always. Sometimes it was necessary to keep the face wet with tears so that the spirits would pity the sufferer, and grant him his request. "I am a poor man. Pity me," is a constant prayer. "Have nothing," the medicine men taught, "and the spirits will come to you." ' Ruth Benedict: op. cit. pp. 58 ff.

[2] Huxley: *Heaven and Hell* (1956) p. 62.

ence. But the matter does not end there. The work of a great artist or a great scientist need not be dismissed because he is a chain-smoker. The chemistry of the physical processes does not necessarily invalidate the *quality* of the result. *It is the quality of the result that is to be judged and not the physical or psychological processes by which it is obtained.* We may, therefore, adopt a suggestion made by Evelyn Underhill[1] that what are often described as 'mystical automations' are 'the *media* by which the self receives spiritual stimulus'; so it may be argued that drug-induced or ascetically induced experiences can be the means by which the human personality is laid open to the suggestion of the unconscious through whose primordial imagery the deeper activities of the soul emerge as conscious recognition of the transcendental.

We have already listed certain features which mystics of all kinds seem to agree upon as being the characteristics of genuine religious experiences; of these we may now emphasize that which says that an authentic mystical experience (whether involuntary or induced) involves a transformation of character – a sanctification – that is both communicable and contagious.

> Psychic experiences, which do not contribute to sanctification, are not experiences of God but merely of certain unfamiliar aspects of our psychophysical universe . . . where there is no evidence of sanctification, there is no reason to suppose that the experience has anything to do with God. It is a significant fact that occultism and spiritualism have produced no saints.[2]

Those who out of their experiences of the Divine are able to lighten the burden of humanity by the achievement of a spiritual buoyancy that helps others to shed the obsessions of ego-centricity, may be judged to have had genuine experiences of the Ineffable, whatever the means employed.[3]

[1] See Evelyn Underhill: *Mysticism* (15th edn 1945) pp. 272 ff.

[2] Aldous Huxley: 'Readings in Mysticism' in *Vedanta*: ed. Christopher Isherwood (1948) pp. 376–7.

[3] One of the most arresting novels in recent years is Georges Bernanos's classic work *Journal d'un Curé de Campagne* (1936) Eng. trans.: *The Diary of a Country Priest*: which gives a peculiarly illuminating account of the devotion of an undistinguished country priest. It is in many ways more revealing than some of the lives written about the Curé d'Ars.

Chapter XII

SOME CONTEMPORARY VIEWPOINTS

In this final chapter we are concerned to discuss the psychological relationship of Group and Individual in so far as this affects the religious life of the individual believer; the possible relevance to religion of extra-cerebral explanations of the relation of body and mind; and the psychology of the individual and his beliefs.

The Group and the Individual

According to Freud, 'group psychology is concerned with the individual man as a member of a race, of a nation, of a caste, of a profession, of an institution, or as a component part of a crowd of people who have been organised into a group at some particular time for some definite purpose';[1] but he went on to offer an explanation of this relationship that is highly relevant to religious groups. This explanation is all the more important because some psychologists have assumed that the existence of a group depends upon the operation of a 'social instinct', but this assumption is not well founded since a 'social instinct' is not an instinct in the primary sense, but a development of the parental instinct. Other writers[2] have advanced the theory that the group possesses a mind whose heterogeneous elements cooperate in much the same way as do the separate cells of the body. The existence of such a mind, if it were a psychical fact, would explain what it is that makes the individual so susceptible to group suggestion. Further, the powerfulness of group influence over the individual increases according to the degree of organization within the group; the more embracive the organization the more easily do the individual members form a 'psychological society'.[3] Other factors which make for psychological homogeneity are a sense of communal

[1] Freud: *Group Psychology and the Analysis of the Ego* (1922) p. 3.
[2] See G. Le Bon: *The Crowd – A Study of the Popular Mind* (1920).
[3] See McDougall: *The Group Mind* (1920).

purpose, the existence of a corpus of custom and tradition, a sense of historical continuity and, at times, a feeling of opposition between one group and other groups. Freud, however, advanced a different explanation of the factors which hold a group together and enable it to exercise a dominant influence over its members. This explanation is of considerable significance for those religious groups which are normally described as Churches.

Group cohesion arises from and is maintained by the operation of the libidinal energy associated with 'love'.

> We may call by that name the energy . . . of those instincts which have to do with all that may be comprised under the word 'love'. The nucleus of what we mean by love naturally consists (and this is what is commonly called love, and what the poets sing of) in sexual love with sexual union as its aim. But we do not separate from this . . . on the one hand, self-love, and on the other, love for parents and children, friendship and love for humanity in general, and also devotion to concrete objects and to abstract ideas.[1]

This means that the response of the individual to the group is strengthened by the need which the individual feels to be *en rapport* with his fellows. In addition to this emotional *rapport* between individuals and the group there is a libidinal relationship between individuals and the group leader. Freud has emphasized the important part played by the horde-leader in primitive societies, but when we study the way leadership operates in more civilized groups we see that it involves not only an ability on the part of the leader to make acceptable suggestions to the group, but also a strong element of mutual stimulation between leader and led.[2] This libidinal sympathy not only reinforces the general feeling already existing within the group, it elevates the leader to a position where he becomes the social substitute for the hitherto privately held ego-ideals of individuals.[3]

[1] Freud: op. cit. pp. 37–8.

[2] See W. J. H. Sprott: *Social Psychology* (1952) pp. 70 ff.

[3] In non-religious groups the exalted status of the leader in part depends upon personal qualities and in part upon such subsidiary factors as prestige. In many cases prestige is reinforced by such ancillary items as ceremonial garments, uniforms, titles, decorations, wealth and an elaborate *montage*. Few of the great personalities associated with religion depend upon such extraneous factors, although they often are employed by lesser men occupying positions of institutional or sacramental significance. But the renunciation of wealth and social elaborations by prophets, mystics and saints appeals greatly to the religious side of man's nature; the material factors which normally stimulate man's sensual and acquisitive make-up playing a less important part in religion. Generally speaking the qualities which belong to religious leaders and founders are such as evoke the most complex of all emotional reactions – the master-sentiment of *reverence*.

But in addition to enjoying a libidinal relationship with the leader who in a religious context may be greeted as 'the lover of my soul',[1] they who belong to a religious group are themselves as individuals strongly influenced by 'all that may be comprised under the word "love" '. This influence promotes a relationship which concentration upon group activities and the unvarying customs of historical institutions have in the past tended to obscure. Today, as in New Testament times, the relationship between individuals is again being recognized as the core of all forms of religious life, a matter which has been the subject of some brilliantly persuasive thinking in recent years.[2]

I and Thou

If an individual enters into a personal relationship with some other individual so that each ceases to be external to the other, then the relationship is no longer that of an impersonal observer to an 'It' but the relationship of love, of I and Thou.[3] Freud, in the quotation just cited, advanced the view that it is the same element that maintains the cohesion of a group as unites those who would otherwise be strangers to one another. On this point, Buber and Freud are in substantial agreement. Most of us look at other individuals as if we were dealing with *things* and not people. We look round a room and say there are twenty people here (counting twenty 'things') or we describe this man as having red hair and blue eyes, or that woman as obviously having 'no dress-sense' – but all such descriptions are expressive of an observational and not of a personal relationship. We are describing persons not as if they were Thous but Its. Buber's thesis is that in the world of It, the world of objects and things, there is a single centre of consciousness whom each of us calls 'I'. But a radically different situation is brought into being when one 'I' confronts another living 'I' and, instead of reducing him (her) to the status of a

---

[1] 'O love divine, how sweet thou art!
When shall I find my longing heart
All taken up by thee?
I thirst, I faint and die to prove
The greatness of redeeming love,
The love of Christ to me.'
C. Wesley.

[2] 'It seems to me that the re-opening of the question of our knowledge of one another is one of the most hopeful events in the philosophy of our time.' John Baillie: *Our Knowledge of God* (1939) p. 201.

[3] Martin Buber: *I and Thou* (1937).

social functionary or a subject in a psychiatrist's case-book, knows him (her) as Thou. This situation may be expressed in yet another way.

The world of It is the world men try to organize or use for their own purposes, but the world of Thou is a community (that is, a world involving personal communion), a world of personal relationships. It is here that we see a fundamental difference between the ordinary group which is an organization under a leader, and a community in which leader and led are related as persons and not as individuals occupying positions of superiority or inferiority. Buber pointed out that men commonly treat God as an It whose existence they attempt to prove or disprove by methods which imply that God is one phenomenon among many. But God as Thou (and not as the subject of a philosophical discussion) can be known only in a personal relationship.[1]

> The idea of God as the universal Other is, therefore, inherent in the act of religious reflection. It is given in the act of reflection itself, which starts from the actual fact of personal relationship. . . . God is not primarily apprehended as an idea, but in life which is centred in *the intention of mutuality*, as that infinite person in which our finite relationships have their ground and their being.[2]

The question of the individual and religion does not end here. It is not commonly realized that modern life is so highly institutionalized that society can no longer exist as a group in Freud's sense of a corpus of persons united by libidinal impulses, nor as a community of persons (what is properly called an *ecclesia* or church) but as a tightly organized hierarchy of *human objects*. Furthermore, whatever degree of sympathy exists between the members of a group, that sympathy is reduced to empathy if we regard one another as functions rather than as persons; a satisfactory relationship can be established (and, by implication, a real *community* brought into being) only if we learn to see ourselves and our fellows as creatures who are made lovable by

[1] Buber says that Jung recognized 'a reciprocal and indispensable relation between man and God' but that this statement has to be qualified because Jung conceived of God as an 'autonomous psychic content'. Religion for Jung, according to Buber, 'is a living relation to psychical events which do not depend upon consciousness but instead take place on the other side of it in the darkness of the psychical hinter-land – but this is not the relation of an I to a Thou but of an I to the psychical content of its own soul'. See Martin Buber: *Eclipse of God* (1953) pp. 104 ff.

[2] John Macmurray: *The Structure of Religious Experience* (1936) pp. 80–1. Italics mine.

the Divine love.[1] A true I–Thou relationship between individuals and the Divine is the factor that makes a community, as distinct from an organized group, possible. The social factors present in the ordinary group are transcended in any community that is based upon a relationship between man and man, and man and the Divine.

Sobornost

Another explanation of the relation of the individual to the community is to be found in a concept used by Alexei Khomiakov (1804–1860) and by Nicolas Berdyaev (1874–1948) – *sobornost.*[2] The word is derived from the root *sobirat* = to bring together, and it meant for Khomiakov not what the word 'catholic' normally does, universal, but *a community in which all men come together without compulsion or an imposed uniformity in the oneness of the Divine.* This community 'is not a multitude of peoples in their separated individualities, but the oneness of Divine grace indwelling in reasonable creatures who freely submit themselves thereto'.[3] Members of such a community know that 'if one of us falls, he falls alone, but no one can be saved alone. Those who are saved are saved within the Church as her members in unity with all the rest.'[4]

Berdyaev, who was deeply influenced by the Russian novelists, developed this idea, and it is chiefly through his works that the English reading public became acquainted with this concept of

[1] One of the criticisms which Jean-Paul Sartre makes of modern man is that he regards himself and his fellow men as actors playing parts – social functionaries. A waiter behaves as if he were nothing but a waiter; a grocer, a tailor or a policeman looks upon himself in terms of what the public expects him to be, so that the individual thinks of himself as a social type and not as a living person who is free to enter into living relationships with other individuals. 'Society . . . demands that a man limit himself to his functions. There are indeed many precautions to imprison a man in what he is; as if he lived in perpetual fear that he might escape from it.' J-P. Sartre: *L'Etre et le Néant*: Eng. trans. *Being and Nothingness* by Hazel E. Barnes (1956) chap. 2. But a man's nature is not exhausted by the social presentations of function; yet most men imprison themselves and one another within a function.

If we acquiesce in our bonds, we are guilty of self-deception (*mauvaise foi*). It is on the charge of bad faith that Sartre indicts psycho-analysts who, he says, allow their patients to find in the 'unconscious' an excuse for avoiding responsible behaviour. This agrees with an entry in Kierkegaard's *Journal*: 'What I really need is to be clear in my mind what I am to do. . . . The thing is to understand myself' 1st August 1835 (trans. Alex. Dru).

[2] The concept is not original to Khomiakov, since *sobornost* stands in the Slavonic text for 'catholic'.

[3] Khomiakov: quoted by Nicolas Zernov: *Three Russian Prophets* (1944) p. 61.

[4] ibid.

sobornost. Berdyaev uses the term in a way that accepts many of the psychological factors usually associated with group life, laying particular emphasis upon the feeling that exists between individuals but insisting that such a sympathy embraces a wider range of affection and a deeper insight than is commonly included under the term 'love'. Unlike those who regard men in society as being bound together by organization, suggestion, gregarious instinct or libidinal emotion, Berdyaev held that men are bound together by the solidarity of suffering and sin. This, for Berdyaev, is the real meaning of *sobornost* – the I and THOU that become WE in an 'altogetherness' of compassion and mutual suffering. This is the true bond of community life.[1]

Extra-Cerebral Explanations

A very different approach to the ways in which man communicates with man has in recent years been the subject of much experiment and discussion. At one time it was felt that these experiments would provide alternative explanations of many forms of religious phenomena and establish an 'inter-subjectivity' that would eventually solve the psycho-physical problems of body and mind.

When Descartes suggested that a small gland in the middle of the brain (the pineal gland) was the point at which mind and body interact, he initiated a series of discussions about the ways in which mind and body are related, none of which has been accepted as a totally satisfactory explanation.[2] Some of these explanations concluded that the mind was dependent upon the physical processes of the brain, but Bergson opposed this view, saying that the brain is only the physical area within which consciousness 'penetrates' matter. Taking his cue from the fact that memories lie dormant in the unconscious, Bergson suggested that memory is a psychical function and that the real purpose of the brain is to act as an 'organ of limitation' preventing too much from being remembered. This point was followed some years later by Professor C. D. Broad,[3] who called attention to two other theories of Brain and Mind, the 'instrumental' and the 'compound'. The first regards the mind as existing independently of the brain. This means that the mind as a 'substance' may not only have been in existence before the physical brain came into being, but that it can continue to exist after the brain has ceased to operate. The

[1] See Nicolas Berdyaev: *Slavery and Freedom* (1943).
[2] For an account of these theories see William McDougall: *Body and Mind.*
[3] C. D. Broad: *Mind and its Place in Nature* (1925).

importance of this theory has been fully appreciated by all those who have been interested in psychical research. The second theory is that the mind is a 'compound' of the body and of some other 'substance'. This other 'substance' is not in itself a mind, but a 'psychic factor' which may continue to exist after the death of the subject carrying within itself for a time those modifications which represent the life-time experiences of the now defunct person. This psychic factor could, Broad suggests, be united for a time with the physical organism of some other person if that person were in an appropriate condition. It is not necessary to emphasize the relevance of these views to those expressed earlier on the nature of the soul or psyche. But one further theory needs to be referred to before we come to consider the subject of Extra Sensory Perception (E.S.P.). It has been suggested that the Cartesian dualism of body and mind should in point of fact be a trichotomy, body, mind and soul. Mind is a factor brought into existence as the result of the soul's contact with the space-time order – though it is difficult to explain how such a contact takes place. This is in many ways similar to Broad's Compound Theory. Mind comes into existence initially as a cluster or bundle of ideas; ideas emerge from the combination of soul and matter in much the same way as water comes into existence as the result of the combination of one part of oxygen to two parts of hydrogen. This means that the mind is a by-product of soul and body, a temporary derivation. These theories bring us to recent researches on E.S.P. What are called para-normal psychological phenomena (such as for example seem to accompany some forms of religious experience) are explained as being due to powers which the mind is supposed to possess and which operate independently of the brain. This extra-cerebral activity of mind is now thought of as manifesting itself in four ways. (1) *Telepathy*, a term used to describe the knowledge which one mind has of what is happening in another mind. (2) *Clairvoyance*, a term used to refer to the knowledge which an individual mind may have of something that is happening elsewhere and of which the subject has received no information by the normal channels of communication. (3) *Telekinesis*, a term which is used to describe that influence which the mind is supposed to be able to exert on matter by means other than the muscular activity of the body. (4) *Pre-cognition* and *Post-cognition*. These terms are intended to refer to a knowledge of events before they actually occur, or to events in the past of which knowledge is furnished by means other than those of memory or the normal records of history. The importance of these activities is such that if E.S.P. proved to be empirically verifiable then we should be in a position not only to offer new explanations about the nature of mind and its relation to the body, but also about many of the abnormal phenomena which have been associated with various forms of religious experience and spiritual activity.

Professor J. B. Rhine and Dr S. G. Soal[1] have conducted for many years experiments with specially faced cards, consisting of five different markings in a pack of twenty-five. These are shown serially to a 'visualizer' in one room and called off by a 'percipient' in another room. As a result of these prolonged experiments it has been suggested that there must be channels of inter-subjective communication distinct from those of the normal senses.

Such experiments have been thought to be of special significance by many persons of repute, but three comments are necessary: first, that there is no reason to suppose that the calls represent anything else than pure guesses, as one might call 'heads' or 'tails'; secondly, that there seems to be some doubt about the legitimacy of applying a statistical law that deals with large numbers to what are necessarily limited numbers of experiments. It is noteworthy also that the most successful performers after some length of time seem to lose their faculty of calling correctly, while the laws of statistical probability are more reliable the longer the chances operate. Thirdly, many accomplished entertainers today are able to put on acts of 'second-sight' which have close resemblances to these experiments, obtaining remarkable 'results' by some other technique than that of E.S.P. The value of E.S.P. experiments is difficult to estimate, but two observations of general importance call for attention.

Professor Gardner Murphy[2] suggests that E.S.P. may indicate the existence of some deep level in the human psyche which confers on man a capacity to be *en rapport* with the whole of space and time. Professor H. H. Price makes the valuable comment that thought is not only powerful, it can be dangerous, for whatever we think about seems to carry with it the power to bring into existence that which was the subject of thought, and if this thought does not in fact actualize, it is because it is prevented from doing so by the operation

[1] See J. B. Rhine: *New Frontiers of the Mind* (1950); G. N. M. Tyrrell: *The Personality of Man* (1946); Rosalind Heywood: *The Sixth Sense* (1959); and contributions by Professor H. H. Price to the *Proceedings* of the Society for Psychical Research.

[2] See Rosalind Heywood: *The Sixth Sense* (1959) pp. 199 ff.

of some stronger thought coming from another person. All of which points to a possibility of great importance for the psychology of religion, but the inconclusive nature of these experiments prevents their results from being applied specifically, although they seem to indicate possible explanations of religious phenomena which are often the subject of considerable doubt or perplexity.

The Psychology of Belief and Unbelief

The nature of belief has been discussed from many points of view since William James delivered an address to the Philosophical Clubs of Yale and Brown Universities in 1896 on 'The Will to Believe'.[1] James described his lecture as a defence of 'our right to adopt a believing attitude in religious matters, in spite of the fact that our merely logical intellect may not have been coerced'.[2] This reference to the 'merely logical intellect' indicates the nature of James's approach. Men are continually confronted with a succession of 'hypotheses', any one of which could become the subject of belief. But only those hypotheses are likely to become beliefs which are judged to be *live*, *unavoidable*, and *momentous*. Hypotheses that are judged to be *live* in cultures which, for instance, believe that the realm of nature is an illusion (*maya*) are likely to be regarded as *dead* by those who live in a civilization devoted to the pursuit of economic prosperity. Furthermore, an hypothesis to be genuinely acceptable as a belief must also be unavoidable and momentous. By *unavoidable* James meant an option that offered no possibility of compromise or evasion, but which forced men to accept or to reject it, while *momentous* refers to propositions which are uniquely important as compared with propositions which are so trivial that it is a matter of no great consequence whether ultimately they are proved to be true or untrue. Belief, then, involves the necessity of choosing between options, but these choices are not made on purely intellectual grounds: 'Our passional nature not only lawfully may, but must decide an option between propositions, whenever it is a genuine option that cannot by its nature be decided on intellectual grounds.' [3] James's assumption that decisions on religious beliefs are made on passional and emotional grounds is not accepted generally today. C. E. M. Joad in his stimulating examination of religious disbelief pointed out that if *the will to believe* is

[1] James: *The Will to Believe – Essays in Popular Philosophy* (1927 edn).
[2] James: op. cit. p. 1.
[3] James: op. cit. p. 11.

divorced from reason it has for contemporary intellectuals no power of conviction.

> Belief in religion comes with a quite special degree of difficulty to persons of my training and equipment living in the middle of the twentieth century. We have been taught to take nothing on trust; to bring everything for judgement to the bar of the intellect . . . faith is hard for us, while the simple unreflecting faith of uneducated persons is impossible. But that is only to say that we have the habits and the outlook proper to educated men in all ages who have been trained to rely upon their intellects. If this were all, it would be of no great value, but there is more to it than that. We are the inheritors of a century of religious doubt. This doubt was never so widely spread or so deeply ingrained. In the circles in which I have moved . . . it is a comparatively rare thing to find an educated man who is also a Christian.[1]

But even if it be agreed that 'intellect can light up only a small area of the universe' [2] those who insist upon the importance of the intellectual factor in belief generally ignore the fact that religious belief is never a purely *passive* acceptance of a proposition that appears to be rationally convincing, but an *active* acceptance of a proposition that carries with it an inescapable *commitment to action.* Some beliefs are of the kind that can be introduced by some such formula as 'I believe *that* . . .' while others are of the kind that require some such formula as 'I believe *in* . . .' [3] The first of these formulas serves to introduce mainly intellectual and rational propositions; the second, propositions which are a basis for living and not merely an addition to an encyclopaedia. Every belief that implies personal commitment involves instinctual and affective elements.

But we have still to answer the question, what is it that causes men to accept as *live* beliefs, propositions which reason can support only to a limited extent? The answer is rooted in the fact that man has a *natural desire to believe.* The instinct of curiosity that causes him to ask questions and to clamour for explanations shows that man has a *natural aptitude* for belief. It may, of course, be contended that man invents particular beliefs with which he seeks to satisfy his instinctual curiosity, but even if this were so in certain cases, this impulse to formulate beliefs springs from the instinctual and affective elements in his nature and not solely from his mental capacities. The urge to believe is indigenous to man. If it were not so there could never be any

[1] C. E. M. Joad: *The Recovery of Belief* (1952) pp. 20–1.
[2] Joad: op. cit. p. 19.
[3] See Leonard Hodgson: *Christian Faith and Practice* (1950) chap. 1.

such reaction as doubt, disbelief and unbelief. When men reject a traditional 'belief' because it is not 'true', they do so – however agnostic or sceptical their outlook – because they hold at least two basic convictions, namely, belief in the existence of a quality called 'truth' and, secondly, a conviction that it is vitally necessary to accept only those hypotheses that can be shown to be true. Those who are disbelievers on one ground, are in fact convinced believers on another ground. This is virtually the position advanced by Simone Weil, who argued that scepticism deeply streaked with belief could often be more vitally real than traditional belief streaked with concealed scepticism.

In this changing world no one is unaffected by doubt or scepticism. Every *live* belief today has its commixture of intellectual doubt – otherwise it would not be *live* – because the centre of gravity in belief, which at the beginning of this century changed from authority to experience, has now changed from experience to intellect. This has been on the whole a dubious change because psychologically it is known that belief is not a purely intellectual *gnosis* – it always involves an intuition (whether it be called 'faith' or a 'hunch') that there is a wider horizon of existence and a deeper profundity of meaning than the mind can explore. This view is soundly based upon the fact that man is a creature whose life is hormically directed to goals which are never fully cognized but to which man instinctively aspires. This aspiration is part of the process by which man hopes to achieve that maturity or 'completeness' for which all men unceasingly yearn.

One of the best expositions of the relation of belief to this craving for maturity or completeness is to be found in Professor H. C. Rümke's *The Psychology of Unbelief.* 'Belief is something which accompanies us in our development and maturity so that the various forms through which belief passes constitute development. Hence, we conclude "Unbelief is an interruption in development."' [1] Belief begins with experience, and experiences, says Rümke, are of two kinds, the cosmic-religious and 'the shapes behind the words' (that is, tradition). The transformation of experience into intellectualized statements of belief is governed by the operation of thought and will-power. But this process is closely related to the development of man both as a species and as an individual. Primitive man was so closely identified with the collective psyche of the human species that,

[1] H. C. Rümke: *The Psychology of Unbelief*: E.T. (1952) p. xi.

like a young child, he was identified with his 'universe', and so was meaningfully linked up with 'the whole of being'. But, again like a young child, he subsequently became aware of himself as a distinct personality, and also aware of a Mystery which surrounded him and his life, and which he later learnt to identify with the First Cause. This recognition of a Divine Cause is accompanied by a slowly developing sense of obedience, a development which can reach its maturity only in the surrender of the self to the Other Self. But progress towards maturity is hindered by many 'interruptions', *interruptions which are*, says Rümke, *among the causes of disbelief.*

Among the obstacles which today prevent man from achieving this essential surrender of the ego[1] are such psychological impediments as narcissism, which plays a prominent part in the excessive individualism of modern man 'who refuses to do anything that is imposed, be it even by God'.[2] Narcissism, in a religious context, is the substitution of one's own ego for the God-imago, a return to the infantile stage when the ego regards itself as the *Primum Mobile.* There are other restraints which make the surrender of the ego almost impossible for modern man. '(*a*) Fear of passivity. (*b*) Fear of dangers which threaten in sexual surrender e.g. the dangerous mother, the fear of emasculation (deriving from the Oedipus Complex). (*c*) The fear of death, probably as a result of (*a*) and (*b*).' [3] Of these, the fear of passivity plays the most prominent part today, since it is motivated by vanity and a feeling of inferiority. But in addition to these interruptions of individual development (which have their parallels in the psychological development of the species) there are today certain social obstacles to belief. The apparent inability of institutional religion to make its message *alive* to men living within the highly technical forms of industrial societies, and the present 'woes of the world', constitute serious obstacles. Why should the individual surrender his ego to a God who must, if He is omnipotent and omniscient, be responsible finally for the present state of society? Belief *in* divine goodness becomes almost impossible when, as Faust put it, 'all life's misery gets hold of me'. But this is to ignore the fact that if man were to surrender himself to the Divine he would find himself delivered from the present materialistic obsession with preparations

[1] This surrender of the ego is directly related to what we have said earlier about the *immolation of the self* in sacrifice. 'Sacrifice by its very nature implies that the sacrificer is giving something that carries the marks of "mineness" ' (p. 148 *supra*).

[2] Rümke: op. cit. p. 44.

[3] op. cit. p. 45.

for racial suicide.[1] The most powerful obstacle to belief (in the sense of belief *in*) today is that men find themselves unable to reach that completeness of personality and breadth of vision which can be achieved only by the surrender of what Ramakrishna[2] called 'the love of the little self', that sacrifice of self which Søren Kierkegaard called the final 'leap of faith', a leap in which the intellect plays no prominent rôle.

If, as is generally agreed, religion begins in experience, then it is necessary to observe that man soon learned that there are some experiences which never yield themselves fully to rational explanation. Hence man's instinctual use of those symbolisms which alone are able to convey the significance of cosmic-religious situations which commonly elude logical analysis. Man's use of primordial imagery should be construed as evidence of his experience of reality. Symbols, says Jung, are in themselves adumbrations of reality.

We are, therefore, entitled to argue that those who try to base belief entirely on intellectual considerations overlook the fact that reality cannot be exhaustively presented by rational means. 'Logic does not help you to appreciate York Minster, or Botticelli's *Primavera*, and mathematics gives no useful hints for lovers.' [3] We need a much broader basis for belief than that furnished by reason or intellect or any other *single* psychological or social factor.

The argument for a broader basis for belief has been well set out by Dr Thouless, who argued that belief involves the active collaboration of at least three elements: (1) tradition, (2) reason, and (3) experience. To which he added the comment that this third element combines three kinds of experience: (*a*) experiences of beauty, harmony, and beneficence in the external world; (*b*) the moral conflict that arises from impulses recognized as good and evil; (*c*) the emotional element associated with the idea of God.[4] But the elements of belief could be arranged so as to form a pattern that might be described as a 'Quadrilateral of Belief' [5] in which the four sides represent the essential elements (1) Institution, (2) Reason, (3) Experience, and

[1] Simone Weil says that the good which God is able to accomplish in the world over any period of time is in direct proportion to the degree of man's own willing co-operation with Him. Without this willingly given co-operation (no matter what it may involve) the goodness of God is 'suspended': see *Notebooks*: Vol. I (1956) pp. 273 ff.

[2] See pp. 114 ff. *supra*.

[3] W. Macneile Dixon: *The Human Situation* (1948 edn) p. 64.

[4] R. H. Thouless: *An Introduction to the Psychology of Religion* (1936) pp. 13 ff.

[5] G. Stephens Spinks: *Fundamentals of Religious Belief* (1961) pp. 175 ff.

(4) Revelation. What Thouless describes as Tradition would be better described as The Institution, since this would emphasize the highly important part played by historical institutions which are responsible for the maintenance of tradition, forms of worship and prayer, and for much that is subsumed under the term 'group suggestion'.

In addition to the various constituents already listed, it is important to emphasize the part played by Revelation in all forms of religion. Psychology by itself can, of course, say nothing whatever about the validity of such revelationary experiences, but it cannot ignore their reputed occurrence. Revelation is normally described as a form of divine communication that is conveyed to man in ways that do not necessarily involve rational processes. But Professor Herbert Butterfield has provided a definition that is likely to win a readier acceptance among those who emphasize the intellectual aspect of belief. Revelation is the means whereby certain events in this three-dimensional space-time world are shown to be invested with a 'fourth dimension'.

> In Christian belief, the scriptural revelation, the Incarnation, the Crucifixion, and Resurrection are events which happen in time, but it is claimed that they have an extra dimension, so to speak, and they carry a fullness of meaning calculated almost to break the vessel that contains it.[1]

The fact that revelation is said to have a divine origin should not exclude it from consideration as a vital element in the psychology of belief. Everything we experience in the course of our lives is not only what it is, it can be psychologically a symbol of *something more*. It is this 'something more' that is the fourth dimension.

Belief is the result of a *living* collaboration of what man thinks, feels, wills, needs, experiences, understands and interprets when confronted with the Divine in whatsoever form it is experienced. The psychology of religion makes its most positive contribution when it shows that religion is that which concerns the 'whole' man, and that the instinctual, affective, conative and cognitive reactions of man to the mystery of existence are those of a creature whose pattern of development down the ages has been that of a human being aspiring after the Divine. The *leit-motif* of human evolution is contained in the words of St Augustine, 'Restless are our hearts until they rest in thee.' The psychology of religion is the psychology of man's aspiration for completeness in the Divine.

[1] Herbert Butterfield: *Christianity and History* (1949) p. 118.

Appendix I

THE NATURE OF THE SOUL

The views which various religions have entertained about the nature of the soul are such as to suggest that man has always regarded the soul as the essential element in his psychical life. Some of the ways in which this concept has been viewed by the ancient religions of the world are set out below.

Egyptian

Ancient Egyptian and Semitic peoples regarded man as a physical frame with an inner 'function' which they associated with the process of breathing, but it was some time before this function was thought of as a distinct entity. The Egyptian concepts of *ka* (genius), *khu* (life and intelligence), *khaibit* (shadow), *ran* (name), and *ba* (soul proper), present a complex picture of the body and its functions. In addition to the Egyptian *ba*, the *ka* was a man's double, a corporeal but invisible guardian genius which accompanied a man through life and then at death preceded the *ba* to prepare a place for him in the heavenly realm of Osiris where it was re-united with the *ba* for all eternity.

The Egyptian ideas had their counterparts in the beliefs of the ancient Persians who distinguished between body, life, soul, form and genius, while much later on the ancient Romans made a distinction between genius and three types of spirit: *umbra* associated with burial places; *manes* the spirit descending to Orcus and *spiritus* ascending to heaven, all being brought to a unity in the *anima* or the mind-spirit.

Hebrew and Babylonian

Hebrew ideas as we find them in the Old Testament are particularly interesting. In the earlier Hebrew records there is no division between body and soul; the 'shades' of the dead in Sheol are not referred to as souls or spirits, neither do the earlier sections of the Old

Testament contain any term by which to distinguish the life of the physical body from blood (*nephesh*) or breath (*rūah*). In spite of the close association of Hebrew and Babylonian ideas it is noteworthy that the Hebrews did not distinguish as clearly between body and soul as did the Babylonians. These latter beliefs are best seen in the Babylonian conception of life after death. The dead lived on in decomposing bodies in a dismal underworld. The soul having some sort of body craves sustenance and so, to prevent the souls of the dead from haunting the dwellings of the living, offerings of food were made to their souls. The belief that the souls of the unsatisfied dead manifested their discontent in the form of whirlwinds and storms arose from the association of souls with breath or wind. Engidu, the Babylonian hero, appears as a whirlwind, whereas the dead Samuel appears as an old man wearing his prophet's mantle.[1] In later Hebrew thought *rūah* refers[2] to the seat of mental activity, but Hebrew thought had no psychological terms with which to describe man's interior life.

Their inability to think of human personality without a body was one of the reasons why the Jews later insisted that the resurrection of the body was a necessary condition for life after death. Jewish thought (despite the influence of Hellenistic ideas) did not accept that distinctive dualism of body and soul which figured so prominently among the Greeks.

The extent to which later Jewish thought was affected by Greek ideas is to be seen in the views of Philo Judaeus (d. A.D. 30). Philo, despite the fact that he was a practising Jew all his life, used the Platonic division of the soul into the rational, spiritual and appetitive, but treated them as functions of the soul and not as constitutive elements. For Philo the soul had two elements, the rational (*nous*) which is divine and immaterial, and the irrational which is corruptible. The divine element had its origin in God to whom it eventually returned.

Rabbinical Judaism, as represented in the Talmud, regarded the soul as being that which exercises a responsible control on the two opposed impulses – the impulse to do good and the impulse to do evil. Dreams were treated as the means whereby the soul could ascend from the sleeping body to heaven to receive a knowledge of divine truths.

[1] Cf. 1 Sam. xxviii. 13, 14.

[2] See such passages as Job xx. 3; Isa. xxix. 24; Ezek. xi. 5 and xx. 32.

Greek

Earlier expositions of Greek views on the soul are now known to be unsound because they were based on the *Iliad* and the *Odyssey* which were at one time thought to be very early expressions of Greek beliefs. Modern archaeology has predated Greek civilization by some two thousand years before Homer. For Homer the *psyche* had no specific function to play during the life of the body, its status was that of a 'shade' in some gloomy abode of the dead. In historical times, Greek thought about the nature of the soul reveals a state of confusion. Pythagoras believed the soul to be a function of the body, but subsequent Pythagoreans regarded the soul as an attunement (*harmonia*) of the various elements of the body. Not until the time of Socrates did the Greeks hear that the soul was immortal. Twice in the *Apology* Plato makes Socrates say that his purpose in life had been to persuade men to care for their souls and to make them as good as possible. While it is difficult to ascertain how much Plato was indebted to Pythagoras and how much to Socrates, it is clear that for Plato the world and every member of the human race has a soul divinely created and indestructible. Aristotle believed that the body and soul had no existence apart from each other, the soul being the body's 'form'. Stoic and Epicurean views constitute a reversion to the earlier beliefs of the Ionian scientists. The Stoics believed that the soul was 'corporeal' and would be dispersed at the next world conflagration, while the Epicureans believed that the atoms which composed the soul were blown away like smoke at the death of the body.

Plotinus and Neo-Platonism

Plotinus (A.D. 204–269) is chiefly responsible for impressing Plato's views about the soul on Christian theology. Plotinus regarded the sensuous life as a sort of stage-play since Plato had taught that 'matter' was unreal; it was not enough to suppress the senses, to know God one must also get rid of the intellect. Intellectual discipline was, therefore, little more than a preparatory stage to ecstatic experiences in which cognition, affect and conation, as well as self-consciousness, disappear and the mystic is alone with God. This doctrine was later to play an important part in Christian mysticism.

New Testament

In the Gospels the term *psyche* in some contexts refers to physical life, in others it denotes the state of a person undergoing emotional stress, while in other contexts it refers to the continuation of life beyond the grave. Three other terms, *pneuma*, *kardia*, and *sarx*, are used to refer (1) to the Holy Spirit and to the psychical life generally; (2) to the intellectual life of man; (3) to the physical aspects of human nature. St Paul, in his use of these terms, differs somewhat from their use by Hellenistic Judaism. *Psyche* corresponds to the body's animating principle; *kardia* is used in an emotional as well as in an intellectual sense; while *sarx* refers to physical or intellectual weakness. St Paul shared the view that the 'body' was a necessary condition for the continuance of personality, assuming that the soul had a *pneumatic* body after the death of the physical body. Speaking generally, the New Testament believes that the soul survives the death of the body, but it shows little interest in the question of the soul's origin or in the manner by which it is related to God. The soul is thought of as both an arena for opposing spiritual forces and also as a unique personality which embraces in one living whole, past, present and future.

Patristic Thought

The Gentile converts who streamed into the Early Church brought with them their earlier beliefs about the nature of the soul. These views were for the most part rejected by the Church Fathers who regarded the physical body as a vital concept in Christian theology, refusing to treat the material world as something wholly distinct from God or as a mere emanation of His Being. The Early Fathers found themselves confronted with two opposed views, the neo-Platonic which believed the soul to be incorporeal and essentially different from matter, and the Stoic which regarded the soul either as an epiphenomenon of matter or as a corporeal entity. In between these two positions there was a diversity of philosophical interpretations, most of which seem to have agreed that the soul is the life principle that animates all living things.

Tertullian in his *De Anima* (c. A.D. 208) regarded certain of the neo-Platonic and Stoic theories as hostile to the Christian view of the body; for him the soul was not incorporeal, having been begotten with the body. On the other hand, Origen (A.D. 185–254) regarded the soul as a sort of 'fallen angel' which, for its past misdeeds, was imprisoned for a time within a physical body and although in continual conflict with the flesh was the life-principle of the physical organism. But the beliefs of the Early Church are best expressed by Augustine of Hippo who, in addition to believing man's inner life exists in its own right, held that man was not a composite creature but a rational soul using an earthly body, the mind (including memory) being a higher function of the soul.

The differences between Tertullian and Origen reappeared in the Middle Ages, but St Thomas Aquinas resolved this opposition by treating the soul as a single life-principle responsible for the spiritual as well as for the mental and vegetative aspects of man's life. Aquinas used the word *anima* as the Latin equivalent of the Greek *psyche*, to designate the soul as that which differentiates the living from the dead.

> That whereby the body lives is its soul. And since life is manifested by different functions on different levels of living things, that which primarily operates every one of these activities of life is the soul. The soul is that whereby primarily we are nourished and perceive with our senses, and whereby we move from place to place; it is also that whereby primarily we understand. For the primary source of our understanding, whether we call it intellect or the understanding, is the soul; soul is [also] the form of the body.[1]

[1] *Summa*: I. 76. 1.

Appendix II

PSYCHOLOGY, THEOLOGY AND THE SOUL

Psychology and theology are both concerned with the 'soul', but what grounds are there for believing that the 'soul' which is the concern of the theologian is the *psyche* which is the concern of the psychologist?[1] If the theologian regards the soul as that entity whose activities are in some measure observable as mental and emotional phenomena, then the psychologist cannot ignore it. And if the psychologist claims, as Jung does, to have discovered in the *psyche* 'the basic raw material of religion' then the theologian cannot disregard the *psyche* without serious results to his own study. The question is, do religion and psychology regard soul and *psyche* as synonymous terms? In Appendix I on 'The Nature of the Soul' we saw that many religions and historical periods did not restrict the activities of the soul to the 'supernatural' but in many cases associated it with such psychological activities as intelligence, will, memory and the like.

A study of the *Book of Psalms* shows clearly that for Judaism and, because of their continued use in Christian worship, for Christianity also, the word 'soul' is concerned with a wider range of activity than that of praise and prayer. It is used to refer to emotion, dreams, nightmares and the like as well as to religious activities. A brief selection of passages quickly substantiates this statement.[2] Wherever the

[1] This subject is dealt with at some length and in great detail by Fr Victor White O.P., in *Soul and Psyche* (1960) pp. 11–31, from which a number of references have been borrowed.

[2] It will be seen that the following quotations from the *Psalms* refer to the soul (*psyche*) in contexts which emphasize emotion, sensation, personality or life-principle.

Ps. vi. 3, 4: 'My soul (*psyche*) is sore troubled: turn thee, O Lord, and deliver my soul (*psyche*).'

Ps. xvi. 11: 'Thou shalt not leave my soul (*psyche*) in hell.' (*contd overleaf.*)

word 'soul' is referred to in the Greek version it is uniformly translated *psyche*, and in the Latin version it is always *anima*. If it be asked whether the New Testament uses the word soul in much the same ways as the Old Testament, the answer is that wherever the Greek New Testament uses the word *psyche*, the Latin translation uses *anima* and the English translation uses 'soul' – showing that in the mind of the translators these terms are to be regarded as synonymous. The following passages show that the word *psyche* in the New Testament refers to psychological as well as to spiritual activities.

Mark viii. 36: 'What shall it profit a man if he gain the whole world and lose his own soul (*psyche*)?'

Matt. vi. 25. Luke xii. 22: 'Is not the life (*psyche*) more than the meat?'

Rom. xiii. 1: 'Let every soul (*psyche*) be in subjection to the higher powers.'

1 Cor. xv. 46: 'The first man Adam became a living soul (*psyche*). The last Adam became a life-giving spirit (*pneuma*).'

A study of these and other quotations of a like nature shows that soul (*psyche*) in the Old and New Testaments refers to nothing less than life itself in its fullest range of interests and activities; man is viewed as a unity, an ensouled body rather than an embodied soul. This is no new conclusion. Tertullian in a famous passage asserts that religion is rooted in the nature of the soul; that the soul of every man is natur-

---

Ps. xvii. 13: 'Deliver my soul (*psyche*) from the ungodly, which is a sword of thine.'

Ps. xxxiii. 18: 'To deliver their soul (*psyche*) from death and to feed them in the time of dearth.'

Ps. xxxv. 4: 'Let them be confounded and put to shame that seek after my soul (*psyche*): let them be turned back and brought to confusion, that imagine mischief against me.'

Ps. xxxv. 9: 'And, my soul (*psyche*) be joyful in the Lord: it shall rejoice in his salvation.'

Ps. xxxvii. 7: 'For they have privily laid their net to destroy me without a cause: yea even without a cause have they made a pit for my soul (*psyche*).'

Ps. xliii. 5: 'Why art thou so heavy, O my soul (*psyche*): and why art thou so disquieted within me?'

Ps. cvii. 18: 'Their soul (*psyche*) abhorred all manner of meat: and they were even hard at death's door.'

This short selection of quotations could be greatly enlarged.

ally Christian – *anima naturaliter Christiana* – and that if man would look into his uninstructed soul he would find there all the basic concepts of Christian belief.[1]

We have, therefore, adequate grounds for holding that soul or *psyche* is the common concern of theology and psychology, and since religion everywhere and at all stages of development treats the soul (*psyche*) as in some sense a life-principle, psychology and religion are concerned with the same field of inquiry though not necessarily with the same set of conclusions.

[1] See *The Writings of Tertullian*: Ante-Nicene Library, Vol. I. p. 37, quoted Victor White: *God and the Unconscious* (1952).

Appendix III

ASSIMILATION AND CONVENTIONALIZATION IN RELIGION

Discussing the nature of conventionalization, Sir Frederic Bartlett[1] argues that 'the greatest stimulus to social change probably always comes from outside the strict limits of the changing group'.[2] But when a group or society adopts a technique, a custom or an institution from another group, the selective conservatism of the recipient group works upon the adopted material until it assumes a form familiar to the social patterns of that group. The name given to the processes whereby alien material is worked up into a socially acceptable form is conventionalization. This is a complex process involving the operation of at least four principles, (*a*) *assimilation*, which is a process by which the new material is incorporated into the cultural patterns of the receptive society; (*b*) *simplification*, which eliminates from the new material elements which are peculiar to the group from which the material came originally, and which are incapable of ready assimilation by the new group; (*c*) the *retention* of certain 'trivial' details which are not apparently essential to the material being assimilated; (*d*) a process of *social constructiveness.*

Amplifying his views on these four processes, Bartlett gives some interesting material of the way in which assimilation worked among the Abrahi, a North American Indian tribe who began, towards the end of the nineteenth century, to engage in industrial and commercial undertakings with civilized American groups. As a result, the new industrial and commercial items referring to quantities and products were assimilated to the ideographic methods previously used by the tribe. Bartlett quotes as a further example of assimilation an account[3]

[1] F. C. Bartlett: *Remembering – A Study in Experimental and Social Psychology* (1932).

[2] op. cit. p. 268.

[3] R. B. Cunninghame Graham: *The Conquest of New Granada* (1922).

of how native Indians who had been converted to Christianity by their Spanish conquerors, were discovered to have secret shrines in which 'the overthrown idols' had been presented with such 'foreign' items as the cap of a Franciscan friar, a rosary and other items associated with Catholic practice. Bartlett concludes that transference of cultural factors from one group to another is not just a matter of social contact because only those features are absorbed for which there already exists a suitable cultural background within the recipient group.

Simplification refers to the fact that when some item of alien material comes to be absorbed in another social setting, it is never absorbed *in toto*, but some single element in the original complex is selected as being vitally representative of the whole complex. Such selective simplification does not operate at once but operates over a period of time, becoming more and more representative as it becomes part of the life of the recipient society. The next process, which is closely associated with simplification, refers to the curious tendency by which groups retain unchanged some trivial, odd or novel element in the matter which has been incorporated into the group life. This tendency seems to show that these particular trivial items are in fact of particular importance to the new group. They may, in fact, possess a profound symbolical significance for the members of the group which is assimilating them.

The fourth element – *social constructiveness* – is of special importance. Every established group has its own particular *trend of development* or, it may be, of regression, so that cultural features received from outside are transformed not only by processes of assimilation, simplification and the retention of 'trivial' items, but also by the group's pattern of development. This tendency welds the elements coming from outside into the general pattern of the group's life, so that such transformations are of a constructive kind.

A particularly interesting presentation of the use of the terms conventionalization and assimilation was advanced by Dr R. H. Thouless.[1] Whereas Bartlett used the term conventionalization to cover four related processes, Thouless used the terms conventionalization and assimilation as names for two separate processes of special relevance to religion.

[1] R. H. Thouless: *Conventionalisation and Assimilation in Religious Movements as Problems in Social Psychology – with special reference to the development of Buddhism and Christianity*: Riddell Memorial Lectures (1940).

Thouless's argument begins with a discussion of the common suggestion that all religions basically teach the same doctrine. This, Thouless says, is not so. What actually happens is that religious leaders and religious movements in their early stages have very different messages, but in the course of time, as the result of social influences, and of cultural and religious exchanges, differences which existed between beliefs and practices in their pristine state, assume something that looks like a standard pattern. Many religions are initially in the nature of a protest against some long-established religious pattern. The protest of Zoroaster as a monotheist against the polytheistic practices of ancient Iran, or the repudiation by the Buddha of the metaphysical teachings of Hinduism, are two well-known examples. But all such protests, while giving rise to new religious enunciations, after a time have a tendency to revert to that particular pattern against which each began as a protest. Religions, however, have yet another tendency, that of drawing into their own stream of tradition elements which belong to alien traditions. These two processes of conventionalization and assimilation were plainly operative in Buddhism and Christianity; both of them reverted to attitudes against which they initially protested – Christianity by resuming certain forms of paganism, and Buddhism by reverting to attitudes basic to Hinduism.

Primitive Buddhism was anti-theistic in the sense that it rejected the existence of 'gods' as objects of worship and sought, in the teaching of the historical Buddha, to present religion as an understanding of the causes of evil and of the ways by which it may be destroyed. In other words, primitive Buddhism was a psychological substitute for theistic religion. Now in the course of many centuries, Buddhism has abandoned its anti-theism and has reverted to the worship of gods, with temples and images, and has placed the figure of the Buddha himself as the supreme god among gods. But this is not to be interpreted as a repudiation of the Buddha's teaching, but rather as an example of man's inherent tendency to offer a greater devotion to the person of the teacher than to his teaching. This may be treated as an example of the libidinal relationship which exists between the leader and the led.[1]

> When we describe as 'conventionalization' the process by which the atheistic healer of souls has become virtually a god to millions of his

---

[1] See p. 175 *supra*.

> followers, let us not make the mistake of undervaluing the religious impulse which leads to the deification. All men's objects of worship demand our reverence, even when these are gods created by men out of strange and unexpected material. . . . If, in the course of its development, Buddhism turned from the ideal of mental self-development to that of religious devotion, and from the abandonment of the worship of gods to worship of the Buddha himself, it is no less true that it turned from his prohibition of philosophical speculation. This also seems to be a development natural and almost inevitable in any religion.[1]

We may, therefore, describe conventionalization as a general regressive tendency in the life of a community. A new teacher may bring a new message but the previous and long established tradition in the end re-asserts itself. Habit in some respects is as strong as instinct itself.

The process of assimilation, the incorporation of elements which belong to an alien source, is perhaps best exemplified by the two movements into which historical Buddhism came in course of time to be divided. Hināyāna Buddhism claimed to be a return to a pristine form of Buddhism which seems, therefore, to exemplify conventionalization, while Mahāyāna Buddhism with its high degree of elaboration is an example of generous assimilation.

These two processes assume various forms in Christianity. Protestantism claims to be a return to primitive or New Testament Christianity, while Catholicism is an elaboration which has absorbed material from many and diverse sources. But Christianity itself, in its practice over the centuries, not only seems to have reverted to pre-Christian modes of behaviour (hence the difficulty of reconciling Christ's injunction to love one's enemies with long centuries of religious wars) but also to have assimilated many alien elements. One of the most eccentric is a religious romance, *Barlaam and Joasaph*, ascribed to 'St John of Damascus', which tells the story of how Barlaam converted Joasaph, an Indian prince, to Christianity. The Indian prince Joasaph appears in the Roman Calendar of Saints, but it is now known that the word Joasaph is a corruption of Boddhisat, the title used for incarnations of the historic Buddha. The Buddha-figure has been *assimilated* into the Church Calendar. Other assimilations include the fact that many pre-Christian images of Mother Goddesses have become figures of the Blessed Virgin Mary, and pagan festivals have become allied with great Christian festivals, hence the date of Christmas. The Old Testament records numerous

[1] Thouless: op. cit. p. 37.

attempts by the Jews to assimilate alien gods, indeed, the work of the early prophets was chiefly devoted to counteracting these assimilations.

All religions exhibit the operation of these two processes. There is a psychological tendency in all men to revert to an earlier state (a psychological regression) and also to assimilate material which appears to provide some strengthening of that devotion which all men feel to Powers greater than anything they know on the level of daily existence.

Appendix IV

ONTOGENESIS AND PHYLOGENESIS AND THE THEORY OF RECAPITULATION

The study of man's development as an *individual*, generally known as Ontogeny, shows that this development is closely related to man's development as a species, the study of which is known as Phylogeny. This relationship between the development of the individual and the species is based on the theory of evolution.

> Ontogeny discloses the remarkable fact that every one of these higher forms, in its individual life-history, passes through a broadly corresponding series, of which the first stage is likewise a single cell, the fertilized ovum. Palaeontology, as interpreted by Evolution, teaches the further striking fact that what is thus true of the individual's history holds likewise for the history of the race, which began in the farthest aeons with the simplest forms, and progresses through ever higher forms, till it culminated, mentally and spiritually, in man.[1]

The theory that the phylogenetic development of the species is repeated, at a vastly increased tempo, in the ontogenetic development of the individual was used by Professor Hall as the basis of a theory of psychological recapitulation. Hall drew attention to the development of children and claimed that their successive levels of behaviour are an ontogenetic recapitulation of the various levels of racial development, or as Nunn put it:

> Professor Stanley Hall . . . bids us see in our little civilized barbarians between the ages of eight and twelve, with their stable bodily form and obstinate good health, and their curious passions for independent life, a clear reaffirmation of a pigmoid stage in human evolution, which still has representatives in the Bushmen and the little people of the Congo forests.[2]

[1] J. Y. Simpson: 'Biology': article in *E.R.E.* Vol. 2. p. 624 a and b.
[2] T. P. Nunn: *Education – Data and First Principles*: London (1941) p. 44.

That the life of the child is a recapitulation of phylogenetic levels of development is also urged by Murphy, who says that many of the athletic games and sports of modern men are examples on the adult level of 'reversion' to the hunting open-air savage. There is a subtle pleasure to be derived from this return to the primitive.[1] Even the toys which children use today have a value from the recapitulatory standpoint. As Professor Jane Harrison observed: 'A child's toys in antiquity were apt to be much more than mere playthings. They were charms inductive of good, prophylactic against evil influences.'[2] Today a child's toys often assume a psychological importance far beyond their value as playthings. A child may not be able to sleep unless accompanied by a favourite teddy-bear, and it is clear that in this and other respects the child's relationship to a toy is often that of the primitive's to some prophylactic charm. The psychology of children and primitives is alike in so many respects, that the way children behave, think and dream throws light on the psychology of primitive peoples and also on the development of the thought processes of the race. Piaget distinguished between a non-logical or prelogical state of thought in children, a distinction which bears a close resemblance to the pre-logical state which Durkheim and Lévy-Bruhl said distinguished the intellectual life of primitive peoples. Childhood is characterized, as is dream-life, by a high degree of imaginative activity. The apparently endless ability of children to indulge in story-telling is closely related to the importance of the myth in early stages of human development.

In its first years the growing child tends to identify himself with his environment and this is connected with his emotional life, so that the way he feels towards things is manifested in phantasy-activity. In this respect the waking-life and the dream-life of children are almost indistinguishable. The figures in children's fairy-stories, ogres, giants, cruel witches, malignant sisters and stepmothers, as well as fearsome monsters, are 'familiar' to the child before he actually meets them in his story-books, because these are the forms in which the child appears naturally to express his emotions, and in this respect the witch-craft, mysteries and myths of primitive peoples exhibit the same general features.

The child's interest in his environment is not at first much concerned with the 'natural' world. In so far as children are interested it

[1] See John Murphy: *Primitive Man – His Essential Quest*: Oxford (1927).

[2] J. E. Harrison: *Themis*: Cambridge (1927) p. 17 n.

appears to be in those aspects which agree most nearly with the phantasy creations of its own mind. This capacity to create in phantasy a world as vivid as, even more than, the external world, partly explains the child's strange concept of himself as *primum mobile*. The adult concept of 'cause' seems to make no impression upon the child-mind except in so far as the child conceives himself to be 'cause'. This joy of being 'cause' is, of course, connected with the general level of phantastic creativity, in which he attributes to himself powers quite unrelated to the actual facts of the situation. These early 'causative' phases lead on to those which are to be found in animism in which powers, general or particular, are attributed to inanimate objects, and the stage is thus set for a belief in magic and finally in a differentiated apprehension of 'cause' as dependent upon the will of an agent. The power to invent imaginary companions may be treated as a parallel to the belief in spirits and fetiches, tribal guardians, guardian angels and so forth, all of which corresponds to the developments we have already noted when dealing with the various stages of religion in its early forms.

* * *

Freud's use of the ontogenetic and phylogenetic relationship enabled him to show that there is a relationship between certain mental states of fixation leading to arrests in the development of the individual and possible arrests in the development of the race. We have already had occasion to refer to 'pauses' and periods of latency in the history of the race, as well as to regressions at certain stages. It would not, therefore, be a matter for any surprise that such regressions, fixations and mutations should, under suitable circumstances, appear in the development of individual persons: that is, an arrest in ontogenetic development may be a recapitulation of certain difficulties which were present in the phylogenetic development of the race.

Jung's employment of the recapitulatory theory is connected with his theory of racial inheritance. Since the human species has a remote, sub-human and even animal ancestry, the racial development has levels which correspond to animal existence, to that of ancestral primates, to the large ethnological groupings. Jung held that the individual not only inherits racial experience and racial modes of reaction, he also inherits in his unconscious (that is the collective not the personal unconscious) ancestral man's *interpretation* of his experience.

And these interpretations are contained in those myths, images and symbols by which our forebears expressed their responses to these experiences. The individual in his mental processes recapitulates the interpretative modes of his ancestors without necessarily being aware that he is doing so. This implies that the phantastical thinking of modern man is a condensation of the history of the psychical development of the race.

BIBLIOGRAPHY

The date after each book title refers to the edition from which quotations are made, and this is not necessarily the date of the original publication.

ADLER, A., *The Practice and Theory of Individual Psychology*. London: Routledge (1924)

ALBRIGHT, W. F. *From the Stone Age to Christianity*. New York: Anchor Books (1957)

ALLEN, CLIFFORD, *Modern Discoveries in Medical Psychology*. London: Macmillan (1938)

ALLERS, RUDOLF, *The Psychology of Character*. London: Sheed & Ward (1939)

ALLPORT, G. W., *The Individual and his Religion*. London: Constable (1951)

AMES, E. S., *The Psychology of Religious Experience*. Boston (1910)

AVELING, FRANCIS, *Personality and Will*. C.U.P. & London: Nisbet (1931)

BAILLIE, JOHN, *Our Knowledge of God*. London: O.U.P. (1939)

BARTLETT, F.C., *Religion as Experience, Belief, Action*. Riddell Memorial Lecture: London: O.U.P. (1950)

Remembering – A Study in Experimental and Social Psychology. C.U.P. (1932)

BAUDOUIN, C., *Psycho-Analysis and Aesthetics*. London: Allen & Unwin (1924)

Suggestion and Auto-suggestion. London: Allen & Unwin (1920)

BECKWITH, JOHN, *The Art of Constantinople*. London: Phaidon Press (1961)

BEGBIE, HAROLD, *Life of William Booth*, 2 vols. London: Macmillan (1920)

BENEDICT, RUTH, *Patterns of Culture*. London: Routledge (1946)

BENNET, E. A., *C. G. Jung*. London: Barrie & Rockliff (1961)

BERDYAEV, NICOLAS, *Freedom and the Spirit*. London: Geoffrey Bles (1935)

Slavery and Freedom. London: Geoffrey Bles (1943)

BERNANOS, GEORGES, *The Diary of a Country Priest*. London: Collins: Fontana (1956)

BEVAN, EDWYN, *Holy Images*. London: Allen & Unwin (1940)

BODKIN, MAUD, *Archetypal Patterns in Poetry*. London: O.U.P. (1934)

Studies of Type Images in Poetry, Religion and Philosophy. London: O.U.P. (1951)

LE BON, GUSTAV, *The Crowd – a Study of the Popular Mind*. London: Fisher Unwin (1920)

BORROW, GEORGE, *Lavengro*. London: Collins (N.D.)

BOUQUET, A. C., *Comparative Religion*. London: Penguin Books (1941)

BOWRA, C. M., *Primitive Song*. London: Weidenfeld & Nicolson (1962)
BROAD, C. D., *Mind and its Place in Nature*. London: Routledge (1925)
Religion, Philosophy and Psychical Research. London: Routledge (1953)
BROWN, J. A. C., *Freud and the Post-Freudians*. London: Pelican Books (1961)
BROWN, NORMAN O., *Life against Death*. London: Routledge (1959)
BROWN, WILLIAM, *Personality and Religion*. London: Univ. London Press (1946)
BROWNE, E. G., *A Year among the Persians*. London: A. & C. Black (1950)
BUBER, MARTIN, *I and Thou*. Edinburgh: T. & T. Clark (1947)
Eclipse of God. London: Victor Gollancz (1953)
BULLETT, GERALD, *The English Mystics*. London: Michael Joseph (1950)
BULTMANN, RUDOLF, *Theology of the New Testament*, 2 vols. London: S.C.M. (1952–1955)
Jesus Christ and Mythology. London: S.C.M. (1960)
BURCKHARDT, JACOB, *The Civilization of the Renaissance in Italy*. London: Phaidon Press (1944)
BUTLER, CUTHBERT, *Western Mysticism*. London: Grey Arrow edn (1960)
BUTTERFIELD, HERBERT, *Christianity and History*. London: Collins (1949), Fontana (1957)
CAILLOIS, ROGER, *L'Homme et le Sacré*. Paris (1939)
CARUS, C. G., *Psyche*. Leipzig (1848)
CARUS, PAUL, *Chinese Thought*. Chicago (1907)
CASSIRER, ERNST, *Language and Myth*. London: Dover Publications: Constable (1960)
CHAMBERS, G. B., *Folksong – Plainsong*. London: Merlin Press (1956)
CHILDE, V. G., *New Light on the Most Ancient East*. London: Kegan Paul (1934)
Social Evolution. London: Watts (1951)
What Happened in History. London: Pelican Books (1942)
CIRLOT, J. E., *A Dictionary of Symbols*. London: Routledge (1962)
CODRINGTON, R. H., *The Melanesians: Studies in their Anthropology and Folklore*.
London: O.U.P. (1891)
COOK, STANLEY A., *The Study of Religions*. London: A. & C. Black (1914)
CORNFORD, F. M., *Plato – The Republic*, trans. Oxford: Clarendon Press (1941)
CRICHTON-MILLER, H. C., *Psycho-Analysis and its Derivatives*. London: Thornton Butterworth (1933)
DIDRON, A. N., *Christian Iconography*, 2 vols. London: George Bell (1891)
DILLISTONE, F. W., *Christianity and Symbolism*. London: Collins (1955)
DOWNIE, R. ANGUS, *James George Frazer*. London: Watts (1940)
DREVER, JAMES, *Dictionary of Psychology*. London: Penguin Books (1958)
DURKHEIM, E., *The Elementary Forms of Religious Life*. London: Allen & Unwin (1954)
ELIADE, MIRCEA, *Images and Symbols*. London: Harvill (1961)
Myths, Dreams and Mysteries. London: Harvill (1956)
Patterns in Comparative Religion. London: Sheed & Ward (1958)

ELIOT, T. S., *Little Gidding – Four Quartets.* London: Faber & Faber (1942)
EVANS-WENTZ, W. Y., *Tibet's Great Yogi – Milarepa.* London: O.U.P. (1928)
FARNELL, L. R., *The Evolution of Religion.* London: Williams & Norgate (1905)
FERMOR, P. L., *A Time to Keep Silence.* London: John Murray (1957)
FLÜGEL, J. C., *A Hundred Years of Psychology.* London: Duckworth (1933)
The Psycho-Analytic Study of the Family. London: Hogarth Press (1935)
FORDHAM, FRIEDA, *Introduction to Jung's Psychology.* London: Pelican Books (1953)
FORDHAM, MICHAEL, *New Developments in Analytical Psychology.* London: Routledge (1957)
The Life of Childhood. London: Routledge (1944)
The Objective Psyche. London: Routledge (1958)
FRAZER, JAMES G., *Folk-lore in the Old Testament,* abridged edn. London: Macmillan (1923)
The Golden Bough, abridged edn. London: Macmillan (1925)
The Gorgon's Head. London: Macmillan (1927)
The Worship of Nature. London: Macmillan (1926)
FREUD, SIGMUND, *Autobiographical Study.* London: Hogarth Press (1936)
Civilisation and its Discontents. London: Hogarth Press (1939)
Group Psychology and the Analysis of the Ego. London: Hogarth Press (1922)
Introductory Lectures on Psycho-Analysis. London: Allen & Unwin (1940)
Leonardo da Vinci. London: Kegan Paul (1932)
Moses and Monotheism. London: Hogarth Press (1939)
The Ego and the Id. London: Hogarth Press (1935)
The Future of an Illusion. London: Hogarth Press (1934)
The Interpretation of Dreams. London: Allen & Unwin (1932)
The Psychopathology of Everyday Life. London: Benn (1914), Pelican Books (1938)
Totem and Taboo. London: Kegan Paul (1919), Pelican Books (1938)
FROMM, ERICH, *Psycho-Analysis and Religion.* London: Victor Gollancz (1951)
FROST, BEDE, *The Art of Mental Prayer.* London: Philip Allan (1932)
GALLOWAY, G., *The Philosophy of Religion.* Edinburgh: T. & T. Clark (1914)
GOSSE, EDMUND, *Father and Son.* London: Evergreen Books (1941)
GRAHAM, R. B. CUNNINGHAME, *The Conquest of New Granada.* London: Heinemann (1922)
GRAZIOSI, PAOLO, *Palaeolithic Art.* London: Faber & Faber (1960)
GREEN, BRYAN, *The Practice of Evangelism.* London: Hodder & Stoughton (1951)
GRENSTED, L. W., *Psychology and God.* Bampton Lectures (1930)
This Business of Living. London: S.C.M. (1939)
The Psychology of Religion. London: O.U.P. (1952)

GRIFFITHS, RUTH, *Imagination in Early Childhood.* London: Kegan Paul (1935)
GRISWOLD, H. D., *The Religion of the Rigveda.* London: O.U.P. (1923)
GUIRDHAM, A., *Christ and Freud.* London: Allen & Unwin (1959)
HADFIELD, J. A., *Psychology and Morals.* London: Methuen (1925)
HALL, G. STANLEY, *Adolescence*, 2 vols. New York (1904)
Jesus Christ in the Light of Psychology. New York (1917)
HAMILTON, J. ARNOTT, *Byzantine Architecture and Decoration.* London: Batsford (1956)
HARRISON, J. E., *Themis.* C.U.P. (1927)
VON HARTMANN, E., *Philosophy of the Unconscious.* London: Kegan Paul (1931)
HEILER, FRIEDRICH, *Prayer: A Study in the History and Psychology of Religion.* London: O.U.P. (1932)
HENDERSON, IAN, *Myth in the New Testament.* London: S.C.M. (1952)
HERFORD, C. H., *Joseph Estlin Carpenter.* London: O.U.P. (1929)
HEYERDAHL, THOR, *The Kon-Tiki Expedition.* London: Allen & Unwin (1950)
HEYWOOD, ROSALIND, *The Sixth Sense.* London: Chatto & Windus (1959)
HILTON, WALTER, *The Scale of Perfection*, ed. by E. Underhill. London: J. M. Watkins (1923)
HODGSON, LEONARD, *Christian Faith and Practice.* Oxford: Blackwell (1950)
HOOKE, S. H., *Myth and Ritual.* London: O.U.P. (1933)
The Labyrinth. London: S.P.C.K. (1935)
HOPKINS, E. WASHBURN, *The History of Religions.* New York: Macmillan (1918)
HOSTIE, RAYMOND, *Religion and the Psychology of Jung.* London: Sheed & Ward (1957)
HUBERT ET MAUSS, *Exquisse d'une théorie générale de la Magie.* Paris: Année Sociologique Vol. VII (1902–1903)
Mélanges d'Histoire des Religions. Paris (1909)
HUXLEY, ALDOUS, *Heaven and Hell.* London: Chatto & Windus (1956)
The Doors of Perception. London: Chatto & Windus (1954). Combined edition: Penguin Books (1959)
INGE, W. R., *Christian Mysticism.* Bampton Lectures: London: Methuen (1899)
Faith and its Psychology. London: Duckworth (1919)
Mysticism in Religion. London: Hutchinson (1947)
Personal Religion and the Life of Devotion. London: Longmans, Green (1927)
Vale. London: Longmans, Green (1934),
ISAACS, SUSAN, *Intellectual Growth in Young Children.* London: Routledge (1930)
The Children we Teach – Seven to Eleven Years. London: Hodder & Stoughton (1932)
ISHERWOOD, CHRISTOPHER, *Vedanta*, ed. by. London: Allen & Unwin (1948)

JACOBI, JOLANDE, *Complex, Archetype, Symbol.* London: Routledge (1959)

Psychological Reflections – An Anthology of the Writings of C. G. Jung. New York: Bollingen Series XXXI (1953)

The Psychology of C. G. Jung. London: Kegan Paul (1942)

JAHN, ERNEST, *Religion und Individualpsychologie.* Berlin (1935)

JAMES, E. O., *Christian Myth and Ritual.* London: John Murray (1937)

Comparative Religion. London: Methuen (1938)

The Beginnings of Religion. London: Hutchinson (1948), Grey Arrow edn (1958)

JAMES, WILLIAM, *Principles of Psychology*, 2 vols. London: Macmillan (1901)

The Will to Believe. London: Longmans, Green (1927)

Varieties of Religious Experience. London: Longmans, Green. 36th edn (1928)

JEFFERIES, RICHARD, *The Story of my Heart.* London: Kingsway Classics (N.D.)

JEVONS, F. B., *The Idea of God in Early Religions.* C.U.P. (1910)

JOAD, C. E. M., *The Recovery of Belief.* London: Faber & Faber (1952)

JONES, ERNEST, *Sigmund Freud*, 3 vols. London: Hogarth Press (1953–1957)

Papers on Psycho-Analysis. London: Baillière, Tindall & Cox (1938)

JONES, RUFUS M., *Studies in Mystical Religion.* London: Macmillan (1909)

JUNG, C. G., Collected Works: trans. by R. F. C. Hull. London: Routledge:

Vol. 4. *Freud and Psycho-Analysis* (1961)
Vol. 5. *Symbols of Transformation* (1956)
Vol. 7. *Two Essays on Analytical Psychology* (1953)
Vol. 8. *The Structure and Dynamics of the Psyche* (1961)
Vol. 9. *The Archetypes and the Collective Unconscious*; and *Aion* (1957)
Vol. 11. *Psychology and Religion: West and East* (1958)
Vol. 12. *Psychology and Alchemy* (1953)
Vol. 17. *The Development of Personality* (1954)

Contributions to Analytical Psychology. London: Kegan Paul (1928)

Integration of the Personality. London: Kegan Paul (1940)

Introduction to a Science of Mythology. C. G. Jung with C. Kerényi: London: Routledge (1951)

Modern Man in Search of a Soul. London: Kegan Paul (1936)

Psychology of the Unconscious. London: Kegan Paul (1933)

Psychological Types. London: Kegan Paul (1938)

The Secret of the Golden Flower. C. G. Jung with Richard Wilhelm: London: Kegan Paul (1942)

KELLER, ADOLF, *Die Kulturelle Bedeutung der Komplexen Psychologie.* Berlin (1935)

KIERKEGAARD, SØREN, *Journal* trans. Alex. Dru. London: O.U.P. (1938), Fontana (1958)

KING, IRVING, *The Development of Religion.* New York: Macmillan (1910)

KING, J. H., *The Supernatural; Origin, Nature and Evolution*, 2 vols. London: Williams & Norgate (1892)

KLEIN, MELANIE, *Contributions to Psycho-Analysis – 1912–45*. London: Hogarth Press (1948)
KROEBER, A. L., *Anthropology*. New York: Harcourt, Brace (1946)
KÜHN, HERBERT, *On the Track of Prehistoric Man*. London: Grey Arrow Books (1958)
LANG, ANDREW, *Custom and Myth*. London: Longmans, Green (1904)
LEE, R. S., *Freud and Christianity*. London: James Clarke (1948)
LESTER-GARLAND, L. V., *The Religious Philosophy of Baron F. von Hügel*. London: Dent (1933)
LEUBA, J. H., *Psychological Study of Religion*. New York (1912)
The Psychological Origin and the Nature of Religion. London: Constable (1909)
LÉVY-BRUHL, L., *L'âme primitive*. Paris (1927)
Les carnets de Lucien Lévy-Bruhl. Paris (1949)
Les fonctions mentales dans les sociétés inférieures. Paris (1922)
La mentalité primitive. Paris (1927)
MACDONALD, J., *Religious Attitude and Life in Islam*. Univ. Chicago Press (1909)
McDOUGALL, W., *Body and Mind*. London: Methuen (1928)
Outline of Psychology. London: Methuen (1923)
Social Psychology. London: Methuen (1928)
The Group Mind. C.U.P. (1927)
MACE, C. A., Stout – *Manual of Psychology* revised: 4th edn, 12th imp. London: Univ. Tutorial Press (1932)
MACMURRAY, JOHN, *The Structure of Religious Experience*. London: Faber & Faber (1936)
MACNEILE DIXON, W., *The Human Situation*. London: Arnold (1948)
MALINOWSKI, BRONISLAW, *Sex and Repression in Primitive Society*. London: Kegan Paul (1937)
The Foundations of Faith and Morals. Riddell Memorial Lecture: London: O.U.P. (1936)
MARETT, R. R., *Anthropology*. London: Williams & Norgate (1912)
Psychology and Folklore. London: Methuen (1920)
The Threshold of Religion. London: Methuen (1914)
MARITAIN, JACQUES, *Degrees of Knowledge*. London: Geoffrey Bles (1937)
MARSHALL, JOHN, *Mohenjo-Daro and the Indus Civilization*, 3 vols. London: Arthur Probsthain (1931)
MATTHEWS, W. R., *The Problem of Christ in the Twentieth Century*. London: O.U.P. (1950)
MAYER, ROBERT, *Kleinere Schriften und Briefe*. Stuttgart (1893)
MAYER-GROSS, SLATER AND ROTH, *Clinical Psychiatry*. London: Cassell (1954)
MERTON, THOMAS, *The Waters of Silence*. London: Hollis & Carter (1950)
MICKLEM, NATHANIEL, *Religion*. London: H.U.L. series (1948)
MITCHELL, T. W., *Problems in Psycho-Pathology*. London: Routledge (N.D.)
MONEY-KYRLE, R., *Aspasia – or The Future of A-morality*. London: Routledge (1932)

MOORE, G. F., *The Birth and Growth of Religion*. Edinburgh: T. & T. Clark (1923)
MÜLLER, F. MAX, *Introduction to the Science of Religion*. London: Longmans, Green (1893)
MURPHY, JOHN, *Lamps of Anthropology*. Manchester Univ. Press (1943)
Primitive Man – His Essential Quest. London: O.U.P. (1927)
MURRAY, GILBERT, *The Classical Tradition in Poetry*. London: O.U.P. (1927)
The Rise of the Greek Epic. London: O.U.P. (1924)
MYERS, F. W. H., *Human Personality and its Survival of Bodily Death*. London: Longmans, Green (1903)
NORTHCOTT, HUBERT, *The Venture of Prayer*. London: S.P.C.K. (1951)
NORTHRIDGE, W. L., *Modern Theories of the Unconscious*. London: Kegan Paul (1924)
NUNN, T. P., *Education: Its Data and First Principles*. London: Arnold (1941)
OSMUND, HUMPHRY, and HOFFER, ABRAM, *The Chemical Basis of Clinical Psychiatry*. New York: (1959)
OTTO, RUDOLF, *The Idea of the Holy*. London: O.U.P. (1950)
Religious Essays. London: O.U.P. (1931)
PEERS, E. ALLISON, *Songs of the Lover and the Beloved*. London: S.P.C.K. (1931)
Spirit of Flame. London: S.C.M. (1947)
PERRY, W. J. *The Growth of Civilisation*. London: Penguin Books (1937)
PFISTER, OSKAR, *Christianity and Fear*. London: Allen & Unwin (1948)
Some Applications of Psycho-Analysis. London: Allen & Unwin (1923)
PHILLIPS, C. H., *The Singing Church*. London: Faber & Faber (1945)
PHILLIPS, MARGARET, *The Education of the Emotions through Sentiment Development*. London: Allen & Unwin (1937)
PHILP, H. L., *Freud and Religious Belief*. London: Rockliff (1956)
Jung and the Problem of Evil. London: Rockliff (1958)
PRATT, J. BISSETT, *The Religious Consciousness*. London: Macmillan (1930)
PRINGLE-PATTISON, A. SETH, *Studies in the Philosophy of Religion*. Oxford: Clarendon Press (1930)
RADHAKRISHNAN, S., *Indian Philosophy*, 2 vols. London: Allen & Unwin (1927)
READ, CARVETH, *Man and his Superstitions*. C.U.P. (1920)
RELIGIOUS OF C.S.M.V., *St Bernard of Clairvaux: On the Love of God*. London: Mowbray (1950)
RHINE, J. B., *New Frontiers of the Mind*. London: Pelican Books (1950)
RIVERS, W. H. R., *Dreams and Primitive Culture*. Manchester: John Rylands Lecture (1918)
Conflict and Dreams. London: Kegan Paul (1932)
Psychology and Ethnology. London: Kegan Paul (1926)
RÜMKE, H. C., *The Psychology of Unbelief*. London: Rockliff (1952)
SACHS, W., *Black Hamlet*. London: Geoffrey Bles (1937)

SACKVILLE-WEST, V., *The Eagle and the Dove*. London: Michael Joseph (1943)
SARTRE, JEAN-PAUL, *Being and Nothing*: Eng. trans. by Hazel E. Barnes. New York: Philosophical Library (1956)
SCHAER, HANS, *Religion and the Cure of Souls in Jung's Psychology*. London: Routledge (1951)
SCHMIDT, W., *The Origin and Growth of Religion*. Eng. trans. by H. J. Rose. London: Methuen (1935)
SEGOND, I., *La Prière – Étude de psychologie religieuse*. Paris (1911)
SELIGMAN, C. G., *Anthropology and Psychology*. Journ. Royal Anthropological Institute. LIV (1924)
SELLIN, E., *Mose und seine Bedeutung fuer die israelitische-juedische Religionsgeschichte* (1922)
SHELDON, W. H., *The Varieties of Temperament*. New York & London: Harper Bros (1942)
SILBERER, H., *Problems of Mysticism and Symbolism*. Eng. trans. by S. E. Jelliffe. New York: Moffat, Yard & Co. (1917)
SIMPSON, J. Y., *Biology. E. R. E.* Vol. 2.
SMITH, J. W. D., *Psychology and Religion in Early Childhood*. London: S.C.M. Press (1953)
SMITH, MARGARET, *An Introduction to the History of Mysticism*. London: Macmillan (1930)
SMITH, W. ROBERTSON, *The Religion of the Semites*. Edinburgh (1889)
SÖDERBLOM, N., *Das Werden des Gottesglaubens*. Leipzig (1916)
SOUSTELLE, JACQUES, *Daily Life of the Aztecs*. London: Weidenfeld & Nicolson (1961)
SPEARMAN, C., *Psychology down the Ages*, 2 vols. London: Macmillan (1937)
SPENCER and GILLEN, *The Beginnings of Religion and Totemism among the Australian Aborigines*. London: Macmillan (1905)
SPINKS, G. STEPHENS, *Fundamentals of Religious Belief*. London: Hodder & Stoughton (1961)
SPROTT, W. J. H., *Social Psychology*. London: Methuen (1952)
STARBUCK, E. D., *Psychology of Religion*. New York: Scribners (1903)
STEINER, RUDOLPH, *Eurhythmy as Visible Speech*. London: Steiner Library (1920)
STOUT, G. F., *Manual of Psychology*. 4th edn, 12th imp. revised C. A. Mace. London: Univ. Tutorial Press (1932)
STREETER, B. H., ed., *Concerning Prayer*. London: Macmillan (1931)
SUTTIE, IAN, *Origins of Love and Hate*. London: Kegan Paul (1939)
TAYLOR, H. O., *The Mediaeval Mind*, 2 vols. London: Macmillan (1930)
THOULESS, R. H., *An Introduction to the Psychology of Religion*. C.U.P. (1936)
Conventionalisation and Assimilation in Religious Movements. Riddell Memorial Lectures: London: O.U.P. (1940)
TILLICH, PAUL, *Systematic Theology*, Vol. 1. London: Nisbet (1953)
The Protestant Era. London: Nisbet (1951)
The Courage to Be. London: Fontana (1962)

TOYNBEE, ARNOLD, *A Study of History*, Vol. 1. London: O.U.P. (1934)
TYLOR, E. B., *Primitive Culture*, 2 vols. London: Murray (1903)
TYRRELL, G. N. M., *The Personality of Man*. London: Pelican Books (1946)
UEBERWEG, F., *History of Philosophy*, Vol. 1. London: Hodder & Stoughton (1875)
UNDERHILL, EVELYN, *Mysticism*. London: Methuen. 15th edn (1945)
The Mystics of the Church. London: James Clarke (1925)
Walter Hilton – The Scale of Perfection. London: J. M. Watkins (1923)
VALENTINE, C. H., *Modern Psychology and the Validity of Christian Experience*. London: S.P.C.K. (1929)
VARENDONCH, J., *Evolution of the Conscious Faculties*. London: Allen & Unwin (1923)
WAGNER, PETER, *History of Plain-Chant*. London: The Plain Song & Mediaeval Music Society (1901)
WAY, LEWIS, *Alfred Adler: An Introduction to his Psychology*. London: Pelican Books (1956)
WEBB, C. C. J., *Group Theories of Religion*. London: Allen & Unwin (1916)
WEIL, SIMONE, *Notebooks*, Vol. 1. London: Routledge (1956)
WELLESZ, EGON, *A History of Byzantine Music and Hymnography*. Oxford: Clarendon Press (1949)
WENSINCK, A. J., *The Idea of the Western Semites concerning the Navel of the Earth*. Amsterdam (1926)
WEST, REBECCA, *Black Lamb and Grey Falcon*, 2 vols. London: Macmillan (1955)
WHITE, VICTOR, *God and the Unconscious*. London: Harvill (1952)
Soul and Psyche. London: Harvill (1960)
WHITEHEAD, A. N., *Religion in the Making*. C.U.P. (1926)
WISSOWA, G., *Religion und Kultus der Römer*. Munich (1912)
WUNDT, W., *Mythus und Religion*. Leipzig (1905–1909)
YEAXLEE, B. A., *Religion and the Growing Mind*. London: Nisbet (1945)
ZAEHNER, R. C., *At Sundry Times*. London: Faber & Faber (1958)
Mysticism – Sacred and Profane. London: O.U.P. (1957)
ZERNOV, NICOLAS, *Three Russian Prophets*. London: S.C.M. (1944)

INDEX OF NAMES

INDEX OF SUBJECTS

For Product Safety Concerns and Information please contact our EU representative GPSR@taylorandfrancis.com Taylor & Francis Verlag GmbH, Kaufingerstraße 24, 80331 München, Germany